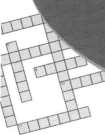

MW00444557

Dr. Pooper's

Activity Book
& Poop Calendar
for Kids

Draw Your Own Rabbit
Start with this example
Now, make your own drawing

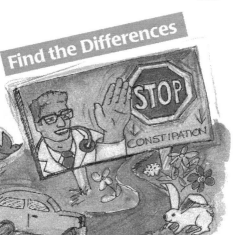

Find the Differences

Match the Shadow

Circle the shadow that exactly matches the snake with the rat in its belly.

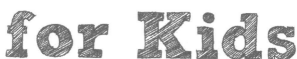

Word Games,
Puzzles,
Mazes,
Drawing, and Coloring
- All About Constipation!

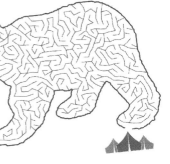

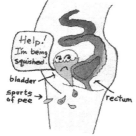

Help! I'm being squished.

bladder

spurts of pee

rectum

WORD SCRAMBLE

These five foods are technically fruits, but most people mistake them for vegetables. Can you unscramble them?

rumccueb

doovcaa

mootta

voile

kpmupni

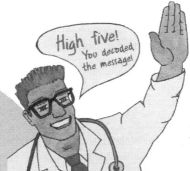

High five! You decoded the message!

DECODE THE MESSAGE

Use the decoder to reveal a message from Dr. Pooper about the best time of day to poop.

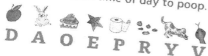

D A O E P R Y V

By Suzanne Schlosberg
and Steve Hodges, M.D.
Illustrations by Cristina Acosta

NEJ
WUQM
AOCMO
QTMOCA
BEKJZIU
ERLZJIWO
UNMHXIAPIV
QWENAPIVF
ICLAFAFF
BLMOEPQAZM
GIXNEAPZM
JUDMTRXLN
TAKRCRQHHE
NVCEPTYSMA
YAWEBPEACH
SITKBPEAEDI
DFFFAPPLET
IADSHGHROW
MFDFGHRBY
RAWBERRY
BERRYWQ
C
D
C
F

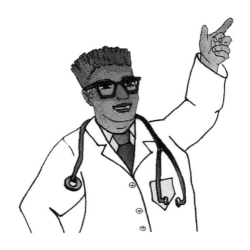

Dr. Pooper's Activity Book and Poop Calendar for Kids, 1st Edition

Book design: DyanRothDesign.com

Library of Congress Cataloging-in-Publication Data is available on file.
ISBN 978-0-9908774-5-5

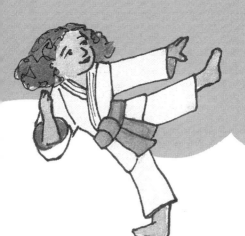

CONTENTS

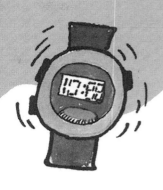

INTRODUCTION

Dear kids and parents,

Welcome to Dr. Pooper's Activity Book and Poop Calendar for Kids!

You probably never expected to buy an activity book about poop and pee, but we think you'll be glad you did.

Constipation isn't fun – that's for sure. But the kids who tested this book had a ton of fun with the puzzles, mazes, games, and drawing activities.

There's something for all ages and interests in this book! Younger artists will love the coloring; older artists will enjoy the Learn-to-Draw pages, created by our wonderful illustrator, Cristina Acosta. Wordsmiths will flip straight to the word searches, word scrambles, crossword puzzles, and Rhyme It! games. Quick: Can you think of four words that rhyme with "floppy"?

The Wordfinder puzzles will challenge 5-year-olds and 10-year-olds alike (and parents, too!). Younger kids can look for the 2-letter words in CONSTIPATION; middle-schoolers will have fun hunting for the 6-letter words. Mom and Dad will find challenges, too!

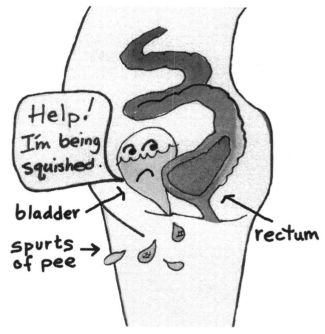

Children who own *Bedwetting and Accidents Aren't Your Fault* and *Jane and the Giant Poop* will recognize the characters and artwork from those books.

The poop calendars at the back of the book make it fun and easy for kids to track how often they poop and what their poop looks like.

We love to hear from kids and parents! Email us and let us know which games you like best and any ideas you have for new ones.

Enjoy the games!

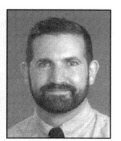

Steve Hodges, M.D., aka Dr. Pooper
shodges@wakehealth.edu

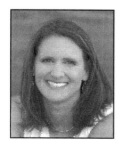

Suzanne Schlosberg
suzanne@bedwettingandaccidents.com

PART 1:
Different Shapes of Poop

Did you know...?

Healthy poop is mushy, like *pudding*, thin snakes, or frozen yogurt. But if your poop looks like rabbit pellets, sausage, or a big log, you're constipated. This means poop is stuck in your belly. That's OK — we'll get it all fixed!

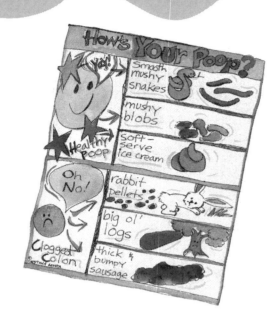

On page 87, you'll find coloring charts to track the shape of your poop every day.

WORDFINDER

How many words can you make out of **PUDDING**?

2-letter words: _____ _____

3-letter words: _____ _____ _____ _____

_____ _____ _____ _____

_____ _____ _____ _____

4-letter words: _____ _____ _____

5-letter words: _____

Word Search: *Shapes of Poop*

Find all these different shapes of poop!
The words go across, down, and diagonally.

Milkshake	Cow Patty	Pellets	Gravy	Hot Dog
Frozen Yogurt	Pudding	Lumpy Sausage	Diarrhea	Walnuts
Thin Snake	Log	Pebbles	Rocks	Fluffy Cloud
Hummus	Mushy Blobs	Marbles	Swirl	Soft Mound

```
K  X  D  N  U  O  M  T  F  O  S  H  B  D  M  U  U  W  Q  Y
V  W  M  Z  N  Z  H  N  P  X  O  E  F  I  P  A  O  D  K  H
C  P  C  H  U  M  M  U  S  T  W  R  Y  A  V  N  D  E  Z  M
C  O  G  X  O  D  D  Z  D  E  O  D  H  R  B  Z  A  K  H  A
N  D  W  L  M  C  F  O  D  Z  A  N  L  R  N  M  B  A  L  D
Q  E  V  P  T  W  G  N  E  S  S  O  W  H  R  L  Z  H  Y  Q
J  R  S  V  A  C  S  N  M  I  I  S  X  E  R  L  K  S  E  G
B  W  B  J  N  T  Y  F  F  D  F  F  J  A  U  L  J  K  N  L
X  A  M  Y  A  O  T  N  L  L  Q  D  O  M  D  H  A  L  P  L
I  L  Q  P  G  D  C  Y  U  F  L  G  P  E  G  N  K  I  R  A
X  N  Z  U  G  Y  G  F  J  R  L  Y  P  A  S  N  R  M  U  G
M  U  R  G  H  T  F  B  I  G  S  F  P  N  T  E  A  B  D  I
V  T  P  C  M  Y  W  W  D  A  G  A  I  C  T  V  I  V  J  T
H  S  T  U  C  A  S  G  U  D  W  H  X  N  X  L  S  J  Y  H
Y  V  P  L  D  A  R  S  Y  N  T  K  R  G  O  L  M  E  M  D
U  H  O  S  D  D  A  B  M  U  S  H  Y  B  L  O  B  S  G  H
S  U  Z  C  T  G  I  H  L  Q  S  T  E  L  L  E  P  X  D  F
D  C  G  H  E  G  R  N  C  E  T  A  P  E  B  B  L  E  S  E
V  O  Z  R  L  I  G  F  G  S  S  V  W  J  M  M  O  H  Q  K
S  K  Q  I  K  F  I  V  R  O  C  K  S  L  Y  U  R  L  W  Q
```

Color It!

Color in your own poop chart!

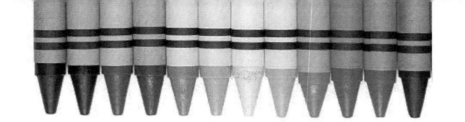

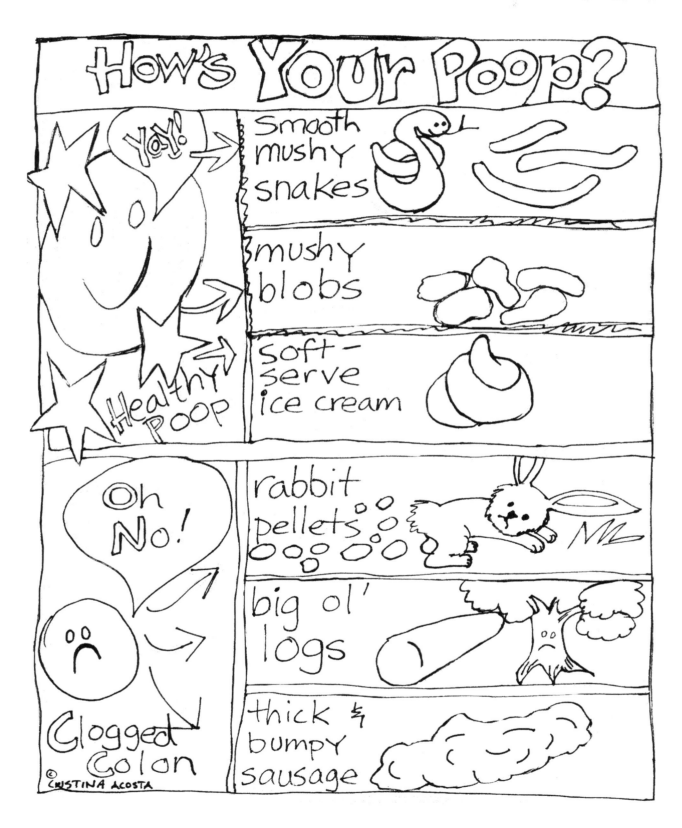

Follow these 4 steps to draw a rabbit.

How to Draw a Rabbit

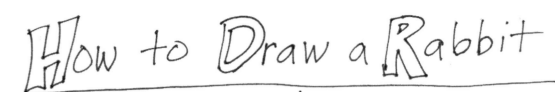

#1

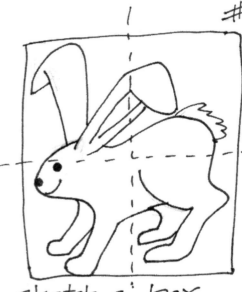

a. sketch a box
b. make dash-lines like this in a t-shape

#2

a. make your own box
b. add the t-shape

#3

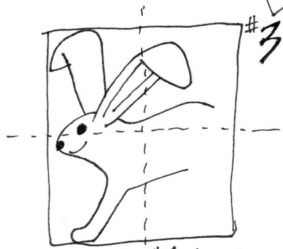

a. look at #1 drawing and fill in each square

#4

a. erase the extra lines

Draw your rabbit here.
Don't forget to draw
her poop, too!

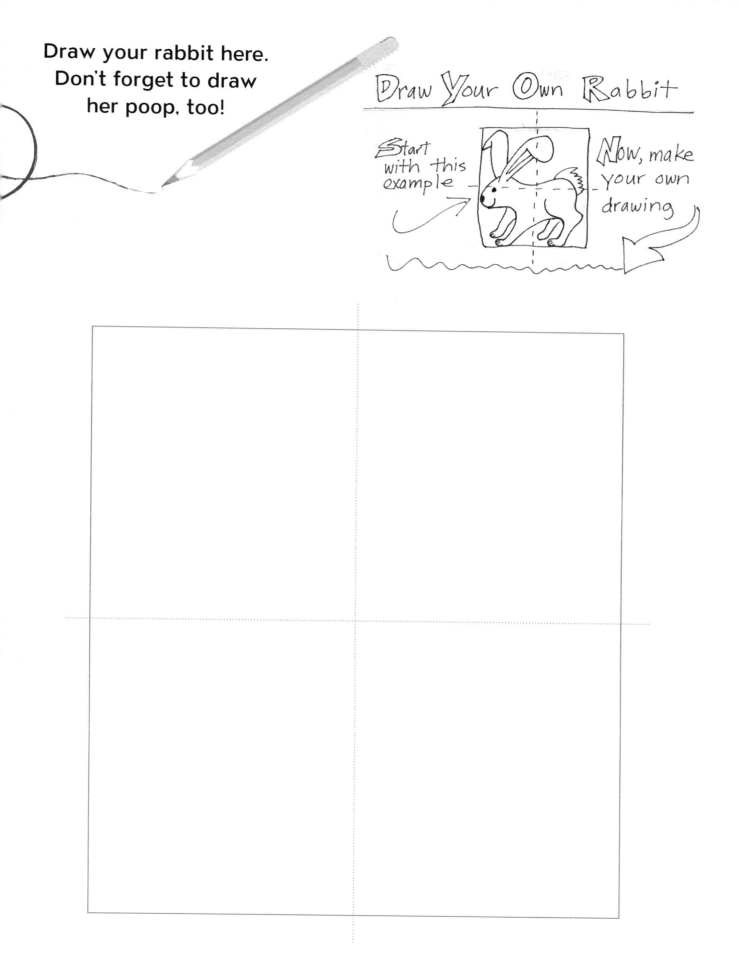

Draw Your Own Rabbit

Start with this example →

Now, make your own drawing

Meet Jane!

This is Jane.
In *Jane and the Giant Poop*, she makes a poop so big that the toilet gets clogged!

When Jane was done wiping she pressed down the lever, but the toilet wouldn't flush — it was a useless endeavor.

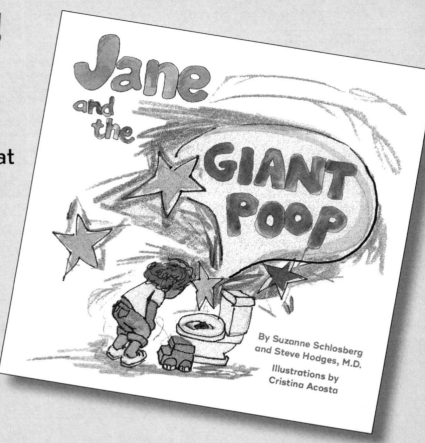

By Suzanne Schlosberg and Steve Hodges, M.D.
Illustrations by Cristina Acosta

Rhyme It!

How many words can you rhyme with **FLUSH**?

_____   _____   _____   _____

_____   _____

How many words can you rhyme with **CLOG**?

_____   _____   _____

_____   _____

Match the Shadow

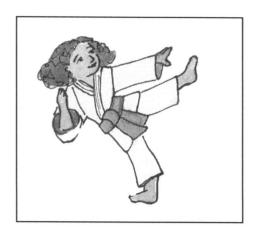

Circle the shadow of Jane that matches this picture exactly.

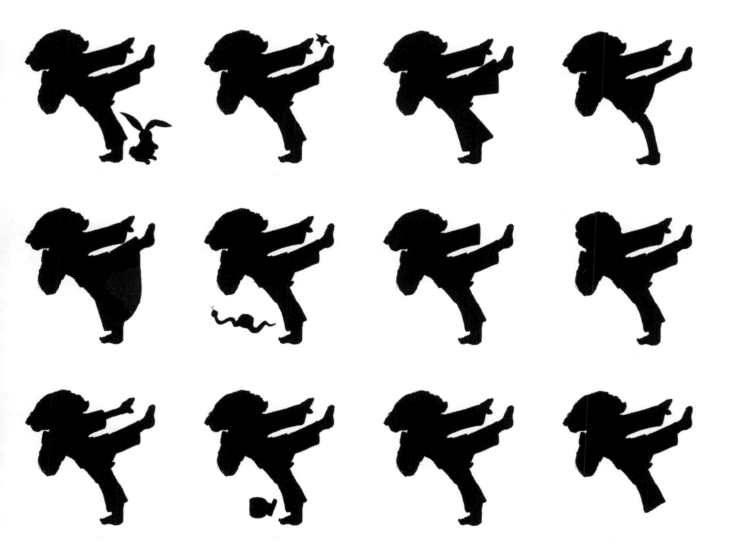

Find the Mystery Words

Each scrambled word below is a different shape of poop. First, unscramble the words. Then copy the shaded letters into the blanks to find the mystery words.

mshuum ___ ___ ___ ___ ___ ___

zefrno uyrogt ___ ___ ___ ___ ___   ___ ___ ___ ___ ___ ___

knase ___ ___ ___ ___ ___

ikmhklase ___ ___ ___ ___ ___ ___ ___ ___ ___

wcotpyat ___ ___ ___ ___   ___ ___ ___ ___

pgdudin ___ ___ ___ ___ ___ ___ ___

glo ___ ___ ___

sbblo ___ ___ ___ ___ ___

sellpet ___ ___ ___ ___ ___ ___ ___

Mystery words: ___ ___ ___ ___ ___   ___ ___ ___ ___ ___

(Hint: This is the best kind of poop!)

WORDFINDER

How many words can you make out of **SAUSAGE** (not including plurals)?

2-letter words: _____   _____

3-letter words: _____   _____   _____   _____

4-letter words: _____   _____   _____

_____   _____   _____

5-letter words: _____   _____

_____

PUZZLE: Jane Tries to Flush!

Cut out the pieces. Glue them onto page 13 in the right order.

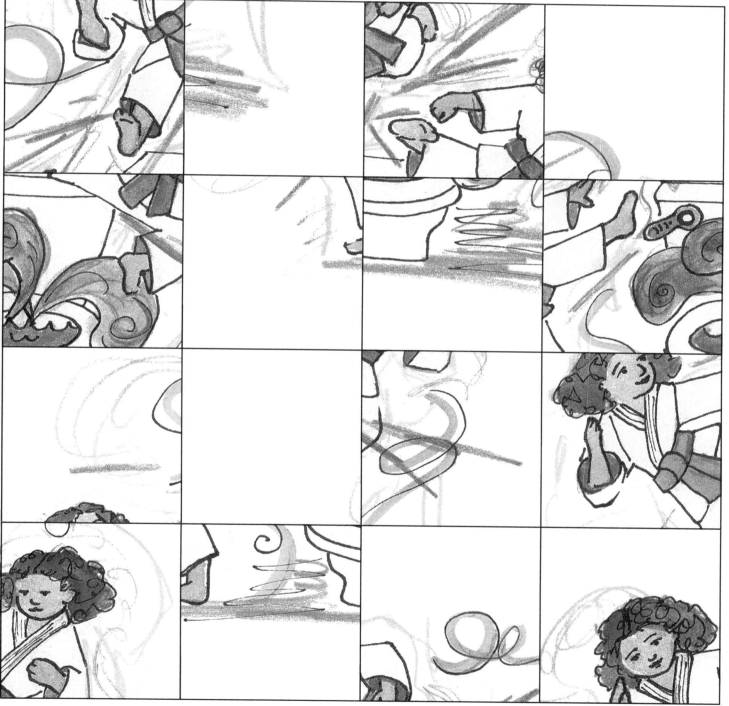

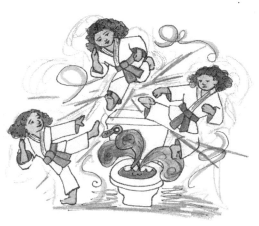

Below, arrange the squares
you cut from page 11
to recreate this picture.

Find the Differences

Circle the 8 differences between these two drawings.

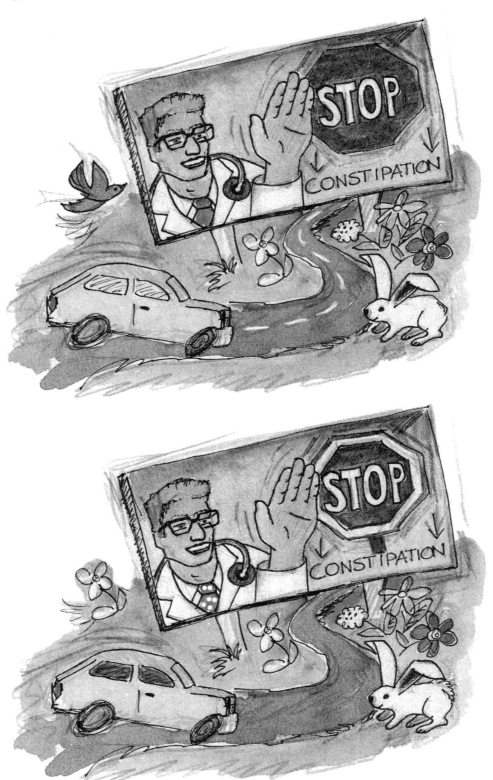

MAZE

Help Jane and her mom find the
way to Dr. Pooper's office!

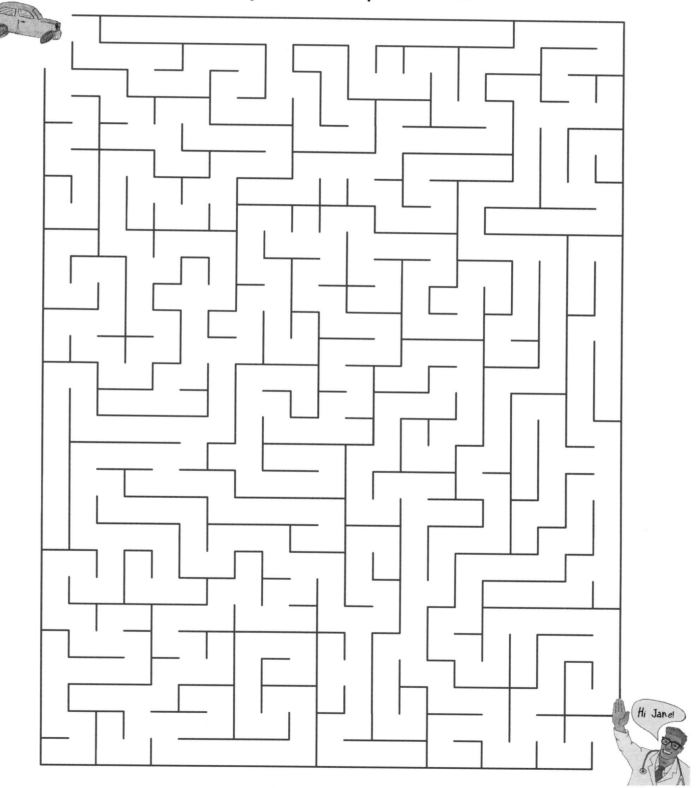

DECODE THE MESSAGE

Use the decoder to read this important message from Dr. Pooper.

D A O E P R Y V

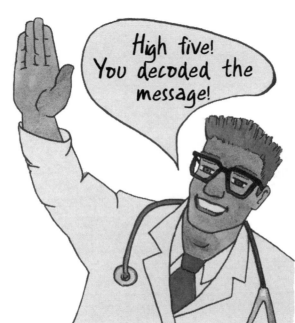

High five! You decoded the message!

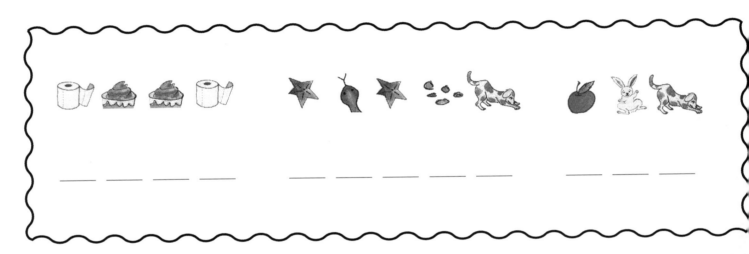

_ _ _ _ _ _ _ _ _ _ _ _

Rhyme It!

How many words can you rhyme with **POOP**?

_____ _____ _____ _____

_____ _____ _____ _____

How many words can you rhyme with **WIPE**?

_____ _____ _____ _____

_____ _____ _____ _____

which is different?

**Jane tells Dr. Pooper that her poops are coming out "hard as a rock!"
Circle the one drawing that isn't the same as the others.**

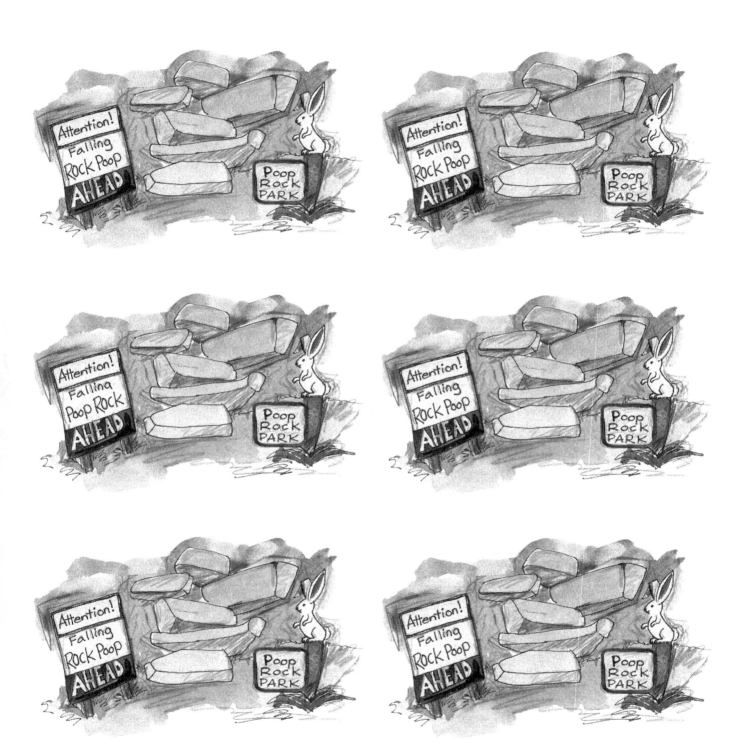

WHICH TWO ARE IDENTICAL?

Circle the two rabbits (and their poop!) that are exactly the same.

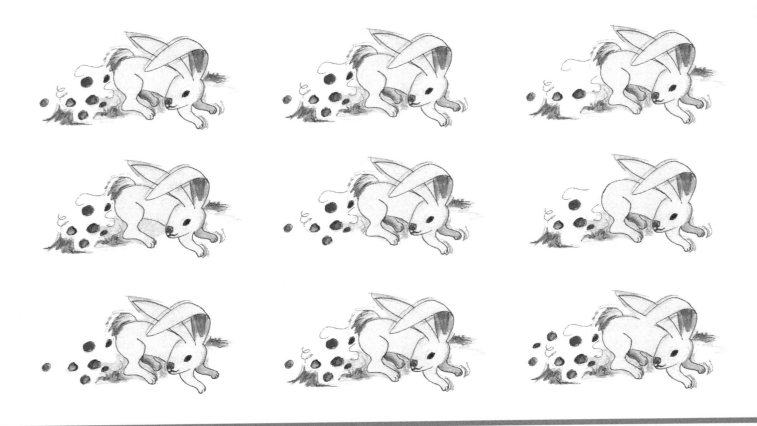

WHAT DID JANE SAY?

Cross out all the capital letters and x's. The remaining letters will reveal how Jane described her poop to Dr. Pooper. Copy the letters in the blanks below.

**W h x C B a L r x Y P d E N
Q V x M R O a x x s Z a D x
S A x X C M r U o x c I A k**

_____ _____ _____

WORDFINDER

Rock-hard poops are a sign of constipation. Poops that look like chocolate milkshake (ew, gross!) are actually a good sign.

How many words can you make out of **MILKSHAKE**?

2-letter words: _____ _____ _____ _____ _____ _____

3-letter words: _____ _____ _____ _____

_____ _____ _____ _____

_____ _____ _____ _____

_____ _____ _____ _____

4-letter words: _____ _____ _____

_____ _____ _____

_____ _____ _____

_____ _____ _____

_____ _____ _____

_____ _____ _____

_____ _____ _____

_____ _____ _____

5-letter words: _____ _____ _____

_____ _____ _____

_____ _____ _____

_____ _____ _____

Did you know...?

Giant poops like Jane's are a sign that your belly is clogged with poop.

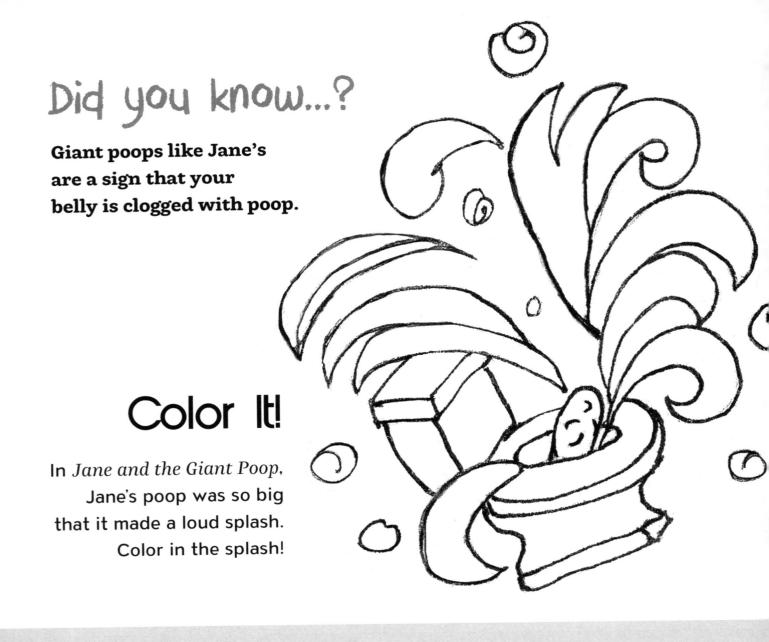

Color It!

In *Jane and the Giant Poop*, Jane's poop was so big that it made a loud splash. Color in the splash!

Rhyme It!

How many words can you rhyme with **SPLASH**?

_____	_____	_____	_____
_____	_____	_____	_____
_____	_____	_____	_____
_____	_____	_____	_____

From "Jane and the Giant Poop"

Jane called for her mom
to come fix the blockage.
"Holy cow!" her mom cried.
"It's a jumbo sausage!"

Jane's dad was in awe
of what Jane could produce.
"That's larger than mine —
snake on the loose!"

Jane inspected the log
and started to wonder
if the family should call
Paulie the plumber.

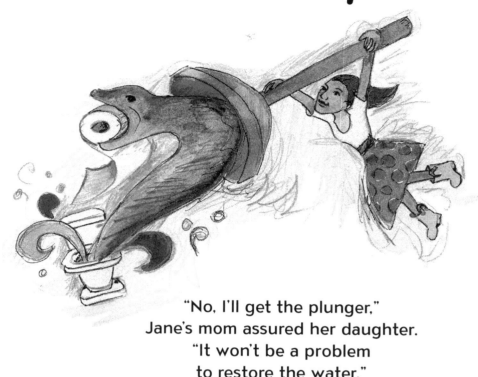

"No, I'll get the plunger,"
Jane's mom assured her daughter.
"It won't be a problem
to restore the water."

WORDFINDER

How many words can you make out of **PLUNGER**?

3-letter words: _____ _____ _____ _____

_____ _____ _____ _____

_____ _____ _____ _____

4-letter words: _____ _____ _____

_____ _____ _____

_____ _____ _____

_____

5-letter words: _____ _____

_____ _____

WHICH TWO ARE IDENTICAL?

Circle the two drawings that are exactly the same.

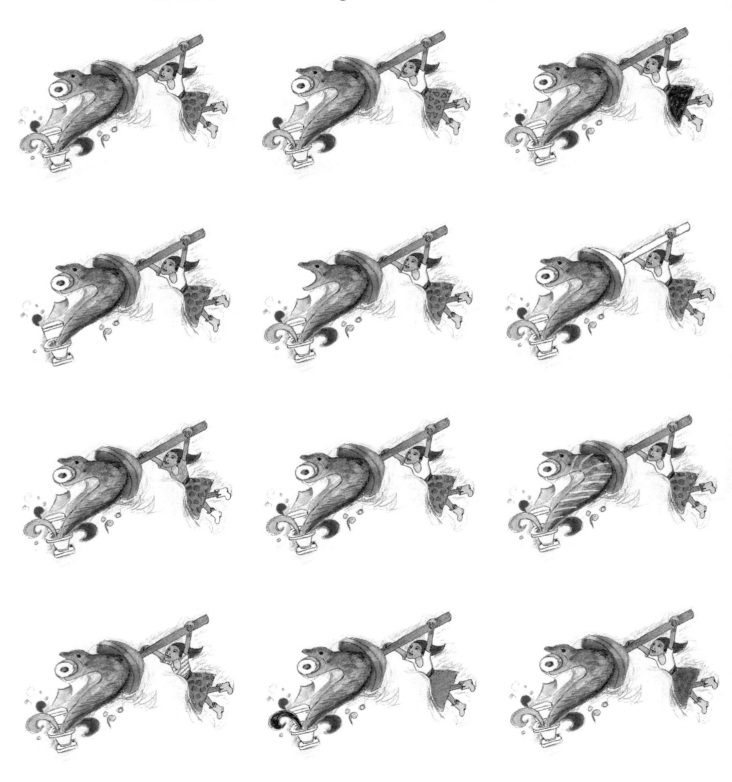

PART 2:
All About Pooping!

Did you know...?

Your body is like a poop factory that never closes! It's always making poop.

Here's how your body makes poop:
After you chew your food, the mashed-up bits travel down a tube called the esophagus and into your stomach. There it gets mashed into smaller bits.

These bits move into a long, twisty tube called the small intestine. The bits your body doesn't need travel to your colon — also called your large intestine — to become poop!

The end of your colon is called your rectum. It's where poop hangs out before you let it out of your anus.

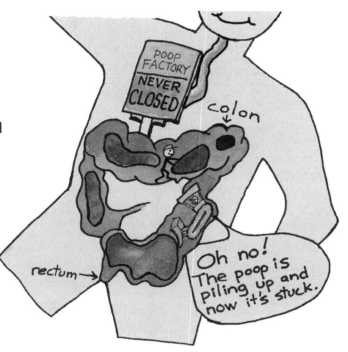

NAME THE PARTS

Fill in the name of each body part involved in digesting food and pooping.

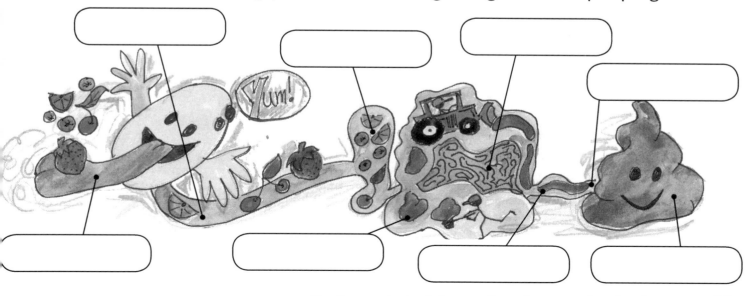

MAZE

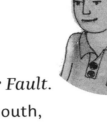

Winding Through Your Poop Factory!

This is Zack, from *Bedwetting and Accidents Aren't Your Fault.*
He just ate an apple. Follow bits of his apple from his mouth,
through his digestive system, and into the toilet.

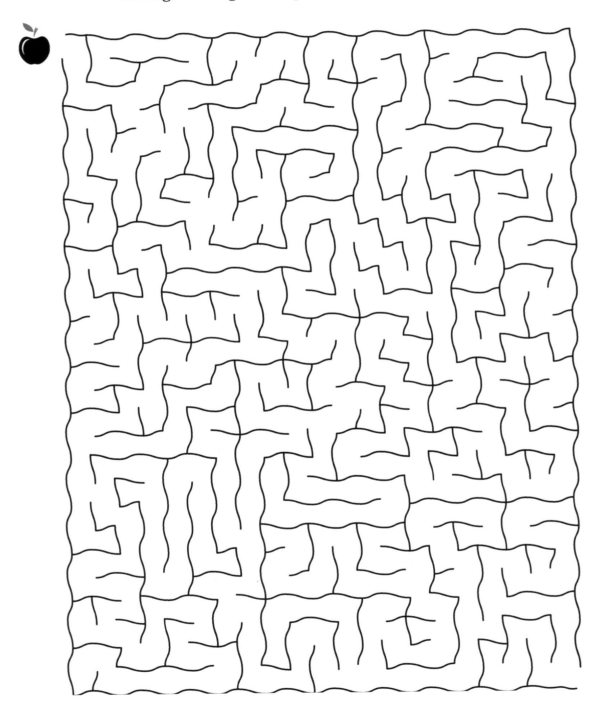

CHANGE ONE LETTER!

Change one letter in each word to create a word related to your digestive system.

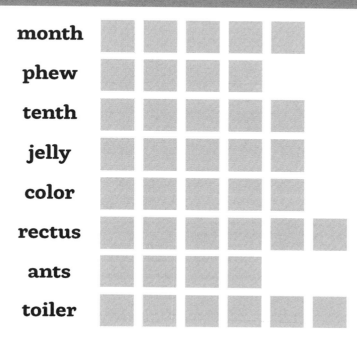

month

phew

tenth

jelly

color

rectus

ants

toiler

Rhyme It!

How many words can you rhyme with **CHEW**?

_____ _____ _____ _____

_____ _____ _____ _____

_____ _____ _____ _____

_____ _____ _____ _____

_____ _____ _____ _____

_____ _____ _____ _____

_____ _____ _____ _____

WORDFINDER

How many words can you make out of **INTESTINES**?

2-letter words: _____ _____ _____

3-letter words: _____ _____ _____ _____

_____ _____ _____ _____

_____ _____ _____ _____

4-letter words: _____ _____ _____

_____ _____ _____

_____ _____ _____

_____ _____ _____

_____ _____ _____

_____ _____ _____

_____ _____ _____

_____

5-letter words: _____ _____ _____

_____ _____ _____

_____ _____ _____

_____ _____ _____

6-letter words: _____ _____

_____ _____

_____ _____

_____

7-letter words: _____ _____

_____ _____

UNCOVER A MESSAGE

Cross out all the lower-case letters, s's and p's to reveal where in your body your poop is most likely to get stuck. Then copy the letters into the message below.

x e r I v q n N o w S P z b
n I r Y S O c b U z P c R S
q i R p E d P S C T u U z M

_____ _____ _____

Did you know...?

If you don't let poop out every day, it starts piling up and hardening in your rectum.

When the poop pile gets super big, it stretches your rectum, the way a snake's belly stretches after the snake eats a rat for dinner!

The big lump of poop is called constipation.
It can give you a stomach ache!

Color It!

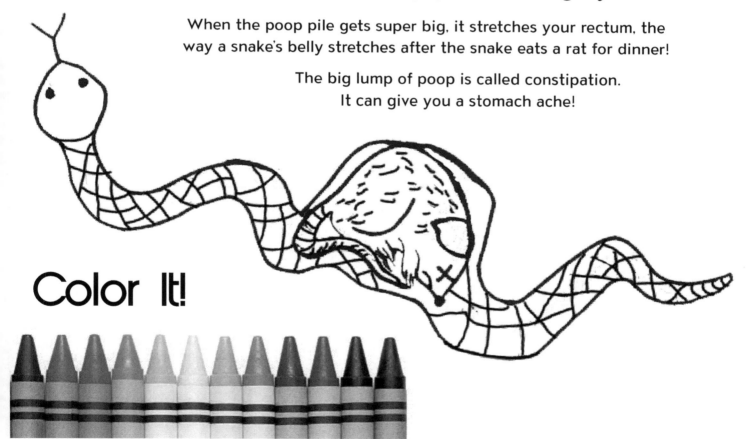

Learn to Draw

Follow these 4 steps to draw a snake.

How to Draw a Snake

#1

a. sketch a box around the snake
b. make dash-lines like this in a t-shape --:--

#2

a. make your own box
b. add the t-shape --:--

#3

a. look at #1 drawing and fill in each of the 4 squares

#4

a. erase the extra lines

Draw your snake here!

Draw Your Own Snake

Start with this example →

Now, make your own drawing

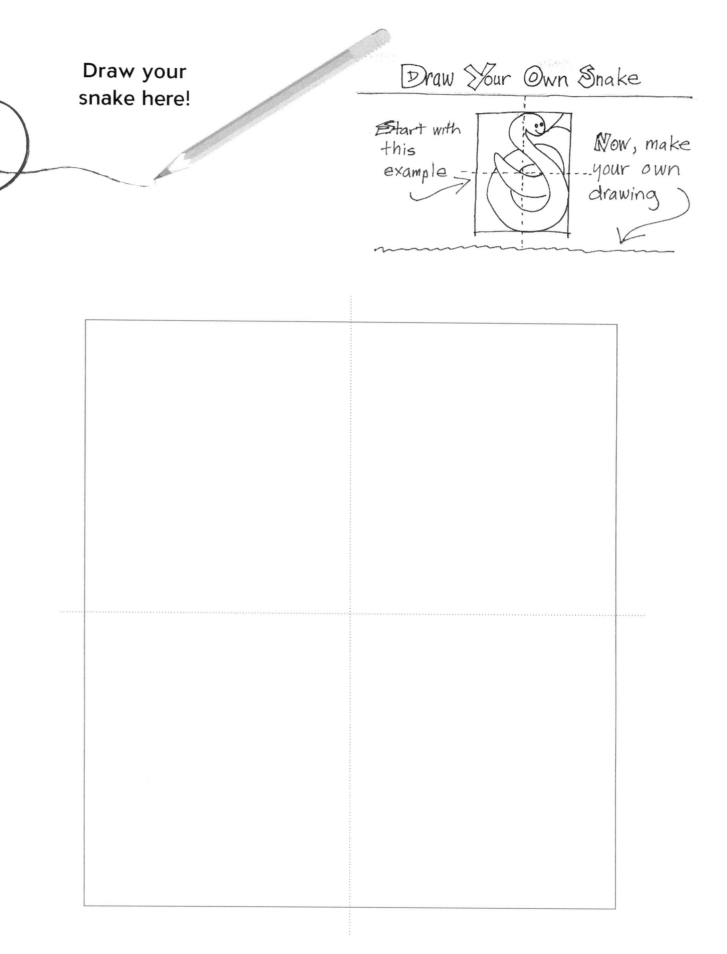

Match the Shadow

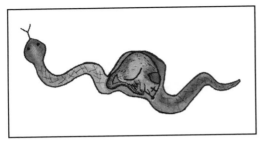

Circle the shadow that exactly matches the snake with the rat in its belly.

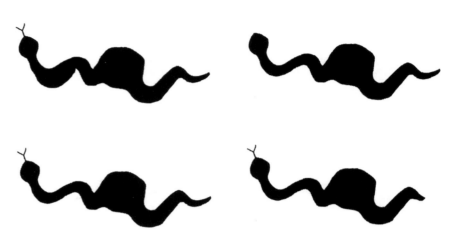

Dr. Pooper says...

When Jane and her mom visited Dr. Pooper, he told them:

"Lots of folks think
a big log is just fine.
However, it's actually
a great big sign."

"It means poop has piled
up at the end of your colon,
in a place called the rectum,
which becomes stretched
and swollen."

"A pile-up of poop
is called 'constipation,'
and happens to kids every day,
not just on vacation."

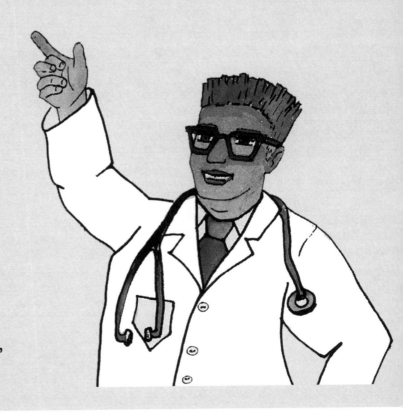

WORDFINDER

How many words can you make out of **RECTUM**?

3-letter words: _____ _____ _____ _____

_____ _____ _____

4-letter words: _____ _____ _____

_____ _____ _____

_____

How many words can you make out of **STRETCHED**?

5-letter words: _____ _____ _____

_____ _____ _____

_____ _____ _____

_____ _____ _____

_____ _____ _____

_____ _____ _____

_____ _____ _____

6-letter words: _____ _____

_____ _____

_____ _____

_____ _____

_____ _____

GUESSING GAME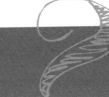

Circle the answer that sounds right to you, and then check your answers in the back of the book.

1) About how big is your stomach?

a) The size of an apricot.
b) The size of a grapefruit.
c) The size of a cantaloupe.
d) The size of a watermelon.

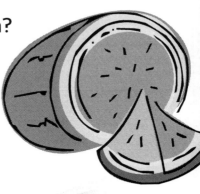

2) How long is your colon, also known as your large intestine?

a) 3 feet
b) 5 feet
c) 7 feet
d) 11 feet

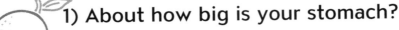

3) How long is your small intestine?

a) 5 feet
b) 10 feet
c) 22 feet
d) 30 feet

4) How long does it take food to get from your mouth, down your esophagus, and into your stomach?

a) 7 seconds
b) 14 seconds
c) 21 seconds
d) 28 seconds

5) After you eat, how long does it take food to get through your stomach and small intestine?

a) 2 to 3 hours
b) 6 to 8 hours
c) 10 to 12 hours
d) 22 to 24 hours

PUZZLE: Driving to Dr. Pooper's

Cut out the pieces. Glue them onto page 35 in the right order.

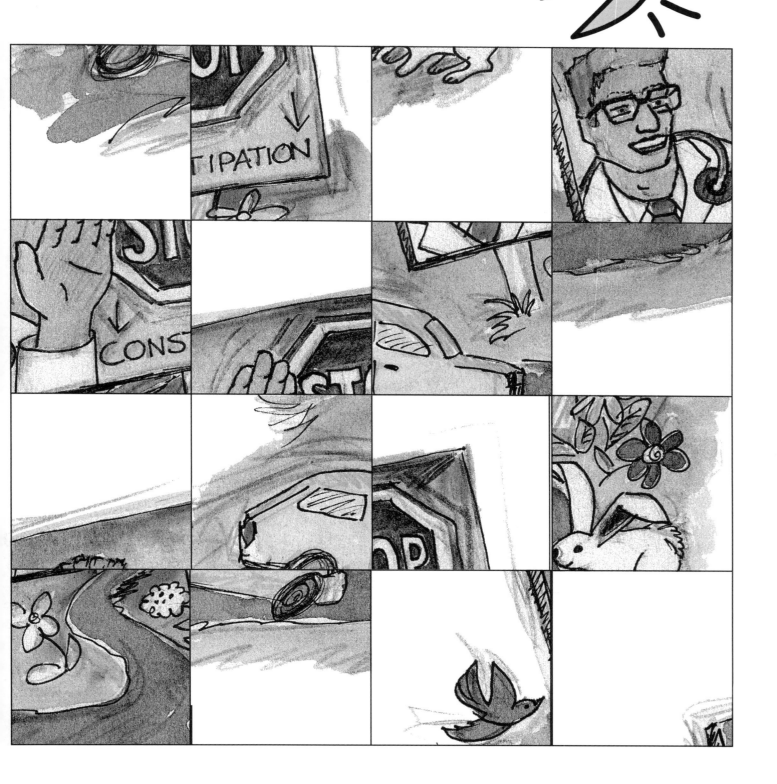

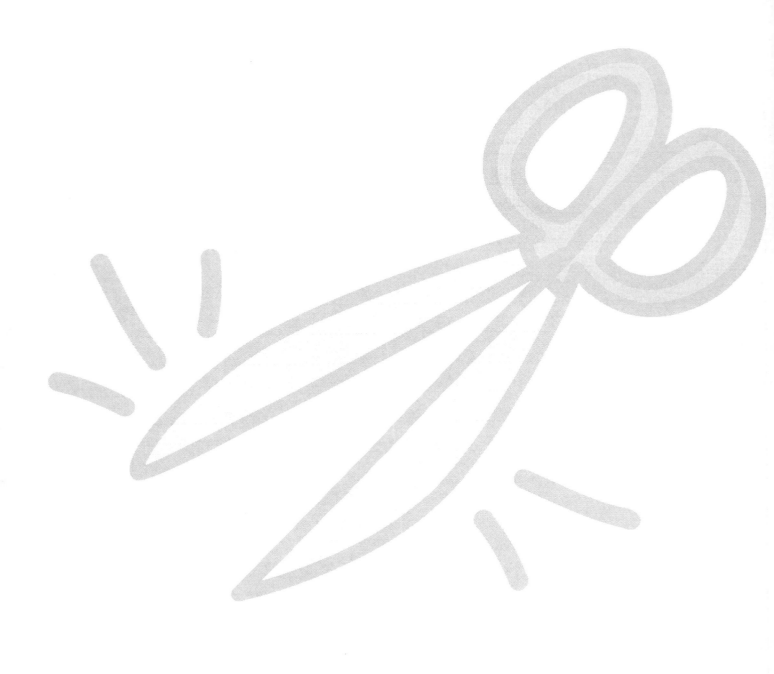

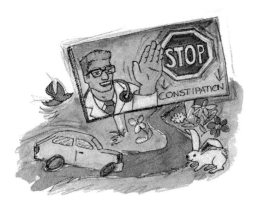

Below, arrange the squares
you cut from page 33
to recreate this picture.

which is different?

Zoe has a stomach ache because she's constipated.
Circle the drawing that's different from the others.

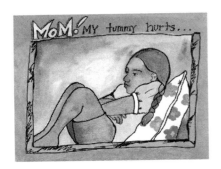
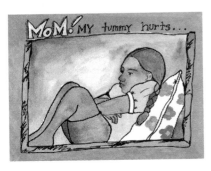
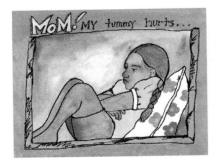
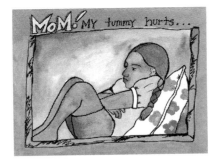
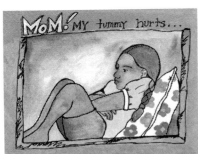
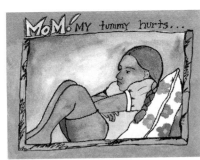

Dr. Pooper says...

There are many ways to flush out poop that's stuck in your rectum. Enemas help the most.

The gentle spray of water loosens and softens the poop that's stuck, the way water streaming from a hose can turn a hard clump of dirt into mud.

After an enema, you feel better because your belly isn't stuffed with poop anymore!

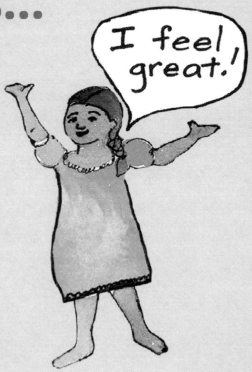

DECODE THE MESSAGE

It can be hard to hold an enema for 10 minutes. Use Morse code to figure out what Dr. Pooper has to say about holding enemas.

B — · · ·
D — · ·
E ·
J · — — —

O — — —
R · — ·
S · · ·

T —
U · · —
Y — · — —

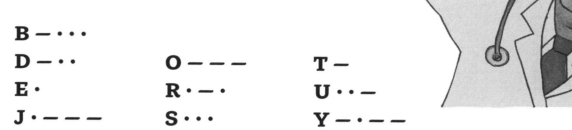

· — — / · · — / · · · / —   — · · / — — —   — · — / — — — / · · — / · — ·   — · · · / · / · · · / —

The slash mark (/) in the message is the space between the letters.

WORDFINDER

How many words can you make out of **ENEMA**?

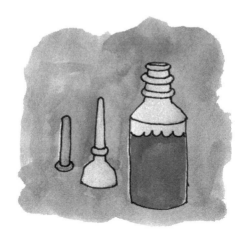

2-letter words: _____ _____

_____ _____

3-letter words: _____ _____

4-letter words: _____ _____

_____ _____

Find the Differences

Circle the 8 differences between these two drawings.

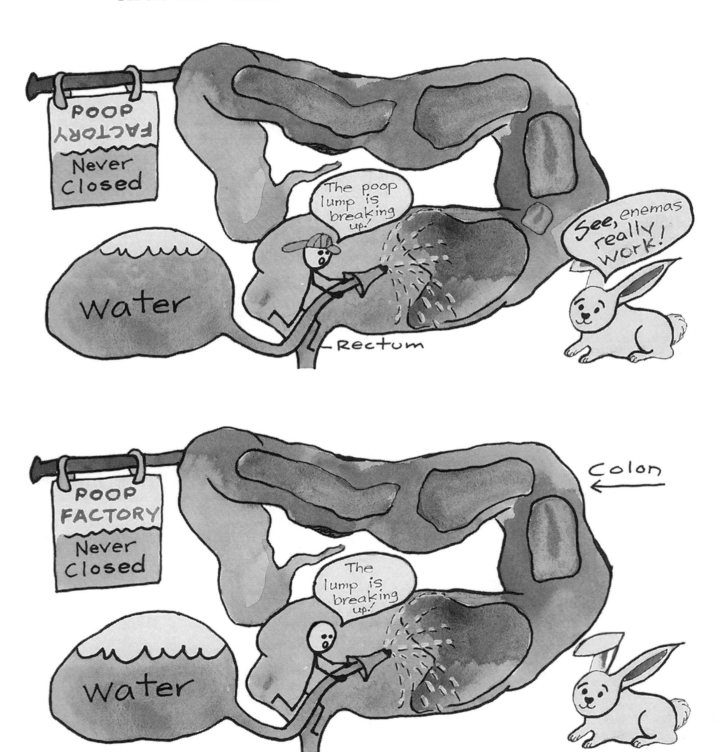

Did you know...?

If you're constipated, it helps to take medicine that softens poop, so it comes out more easily. You can choose from different kinds of "mushy poop" medicines:

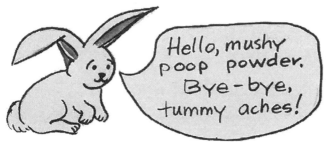

- Powder that you mix with water or other drinks
- Syrup you pour into a little cup or a spoon
- Tablets you swallow
- Tablets you chew

You might need to try different medicines before you figure out which ones work best for your body.

WHICH TWO ARE IDENTICAL?

Circle the two cannisters of mushy-poop powder that are exactly the same.

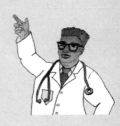

Dr. Pooper says...

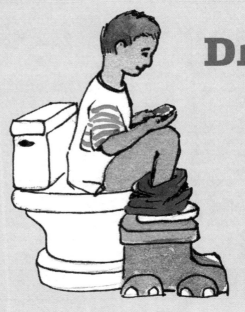

When you poop, sit on the toilet for at least 5 minutes. Don't just hop right off! What if you don't feel like you have to poop? Sit for 5 whole minutes, anyway. You won't know until you try.

DECODE THE MESSAGE

Use Morse Code to reveal a message from Dr. Pooper about the best time of day to poop.

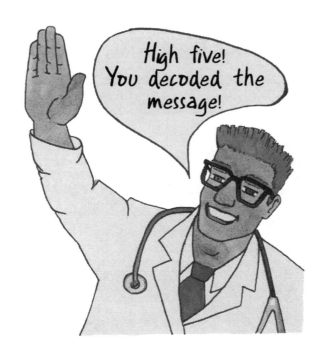

High five! You decoded the message!

A · —	H · · · ·	
E ·	I · ·	T —
F · · — ·	O — — —	U · · —
G — — ·	R · — — ·	Y — · — —

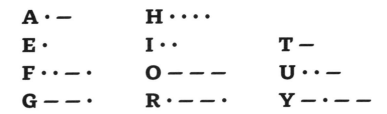

· — — · / · · / — — · / · · · · / —   · — / · · · — · / — / · / · — · ·   — · — — / — — — / · · ·   · / · — / —

The slash mark (/) in the message is the space between the letters.

Did you know...?

Poop comes out more easily if you poop with a tall stool under your feet?

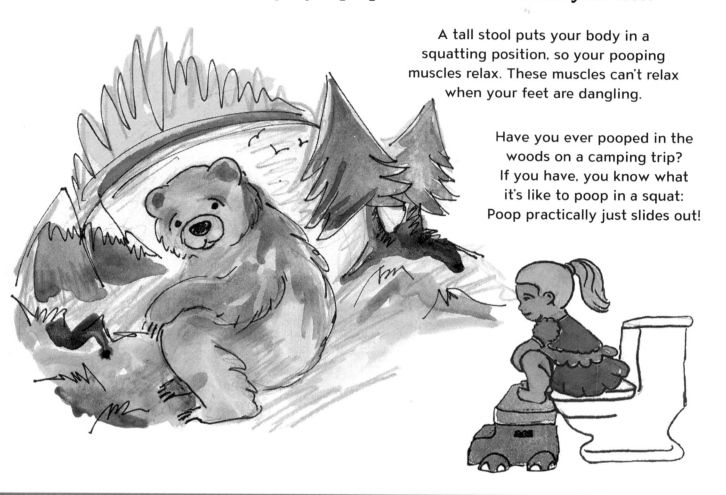

A tall stool puts your body in a squatting position, so your pooping muscles relax. These muscles can't relax when your feet are dangling.

Have you ever pooped in the woods on a camping trip? If you have, you know what it's like to poop in a squat: Poop practically just slides out!

WORD SCRAMBLE

Unscramble the words to learn the 4 rules for perfect pooping posture:

1. Place your feet on a **oslto**

2. Lean **fdorraw**

3. Put your elbows on your **eksne**

4. Keep your legs **trpaa**

Word Search: *In the Woods*

How many forest animals can you find? The words go across, down, and diagonally.

Badger
Bear
Bobcat
Caterpillar
Chipmunk

Coyote
Cricket
Crow
Deer
Dormouse

Eagle
Fox
Frog
Groundhog
Hawk

Oppossum
Owl
Porcupine
Rabbit
Raccoon

Weasel
Wolf
Wolverine
Woodchuk
Woodpecker

```
Q S Q Y V A Q Y Z O H V O F F Y R H T I
K R R B W H F G R O P P O S S U M D F G
C R A O E J Y D R I H E B L E C B M O S
H J C B Y V V Y R O U W P V A R C O X B
I B C I B Q S X Z A U T H Z G I A U F E
P V O A Q I V H L R T N X S L C T Q G A
M T O V A D T A D T R L D T E K E G B R
U M N N O J G H Z M T H M H G E R D E O
N G A H W E A S E L N M W R O T P H H W
K F Q B J O G P I K T Y M Z K G I U W L
S P O R C U P I N E E U D E E R L B O B
P C U R W O L F Q V D P Y B T G L O L Q
F E V C Z K W S M Q K I J U O H A B V D
M P Z Y R H W O O D P E C K E R R C E O
H L I P A O A E O F U F L P V W X A R R
P D W H O V W W X D C L N X E N T T I M
M Y A L D O M Y K G C X I O F R O G N O
J B A D G E R C A S I H Z M A J R Z E U
A C C O Y O T E Z J C N U O G D Z A O S
F F S J Y H S M S I G J S K V K W U P E
```

MAZE

On a camping trip Jane pooped in the woods,
squatting like she does at home with her stool.
Help Jane find her way back to the tent!

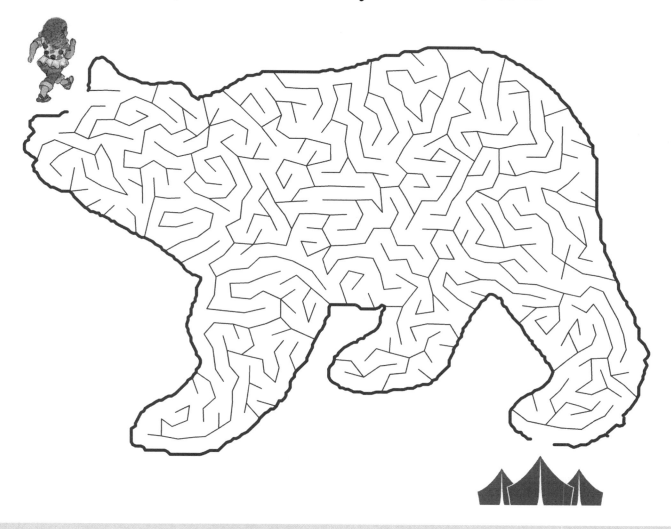

Rhyme It!

How many words can you rhyme with **STOOL**?

_____ _____ _____ _____

_____ _____ _____ _____

_____ _____ _____ _____

Learn to Draw

Follow these steps to draw a bear.

How to Draw a Bear

#1

a. sketch box around bear
b. make dash-lines in a t-shape

#2

a. make your own box
b. add the t-shape

#3

a. look at drawing #1 and fill in each of the four squares

#4

a. erase the extra lines

Draw your bear here!

Draw Your Own Bear

Start with this example

Now, make your own drawing

CROSSWORD: FOLLOW YOUR FOOD!

Use the clues to fill in the puzzle. The words relate to how your body makes poop and pee.

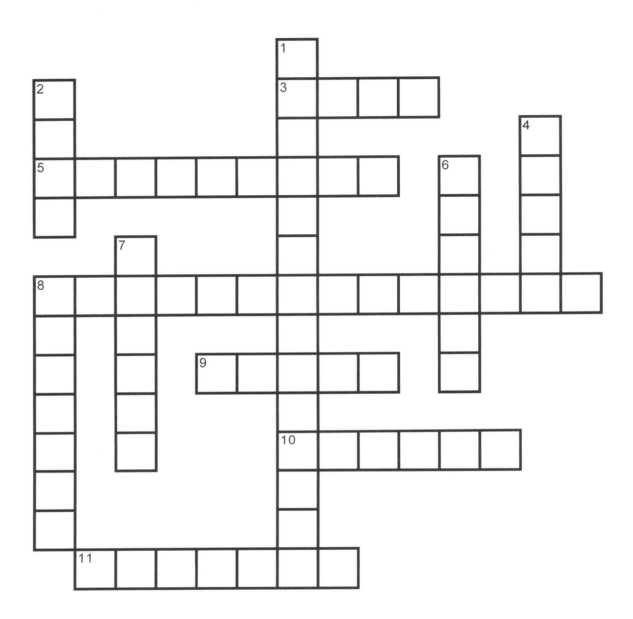

Across:
3 Your body's "exit door" for poop
5 Food slides down this tube to get to your stomach
8 The longest organ in your body
9 Needed for chomping!
10 It moves food around your mouth
11 It gets squished when your rectum is stuffed with poop

Down:
1 Where poop forms
2 You need teeth to do this
4 Another name for large intestine
6 Where poop piles up if you don't let it out
7 Liquid in your mouth that breaks down food
8 Where your food lands after you swallow it

PART 3:
All About Peeing

Did you know...?

Your bladder is a stretchy bag that holds your pee. It's sort of like a balloon.

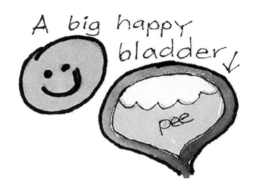

When you eat watery foods — like fruits, vegetables, or soup — or when you drink a beverage, your bladder starts to fill up. When it gets full enough, your bladder sends a signal to your brain telling you: It's time to pee! Your bladder stays big and healthy when you listen to the signal and pee often.

WHICH TWO ARE IDENTICAL?

Circle the two balloons that are exactly the same.

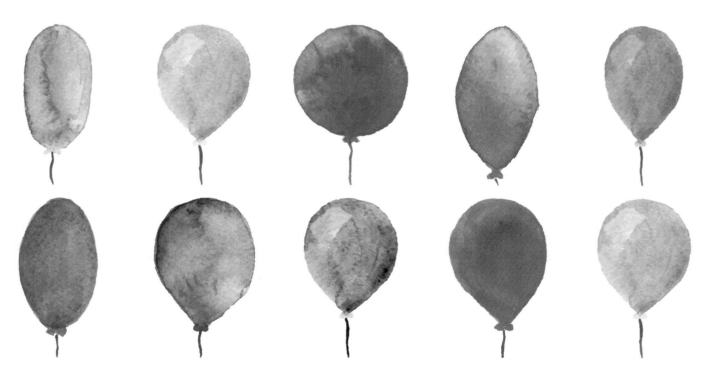

WORDFINDER

How many words can you make out of **BLADDER**?

2-letter words: _____   _____

3-letter words: _____   _____   _____   _____

_____   _____   _____   _____

_____   _____   _____   _____

_____   _____   _____   _____

4-letter words: _____   _____   _____

_____   _____   _____

_____   _____   _____

_____   _____   _____

_____   _____   _____

_____   _____   _____

_____

5-letter words: _____   _____   _____

_____   _____   _____

_____   _____   _____

Rhyme It!

How many words can you rhyme with **BLADDER**?

_____   _____   _____

MAZE

Zoe is playing at the park when her mom reminds her it's been 2 hours since she last peed. Help her find the bathroom!

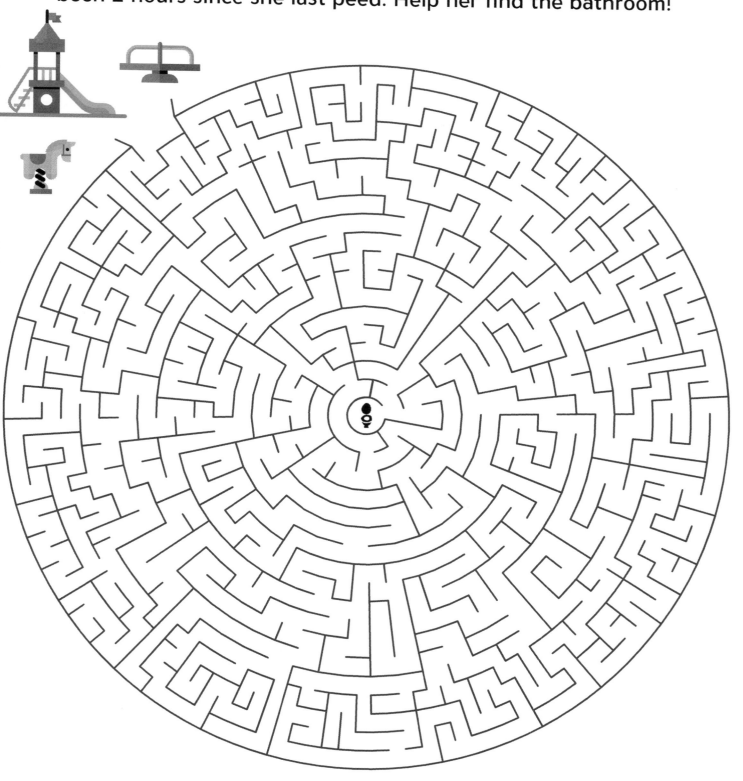

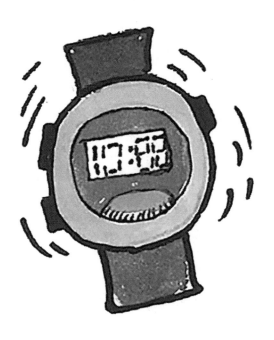

Did you know...?

Your bladder is healthiest and happiest when you pee about every 2 hours.

A potty watch that vibrates will remind you to use the bathroom. Potty watches are great because they don't make any noise!

WHICH TWO ARE IDENTICAL?

Zack and Zoe have matching potty watches. Circle their watches!

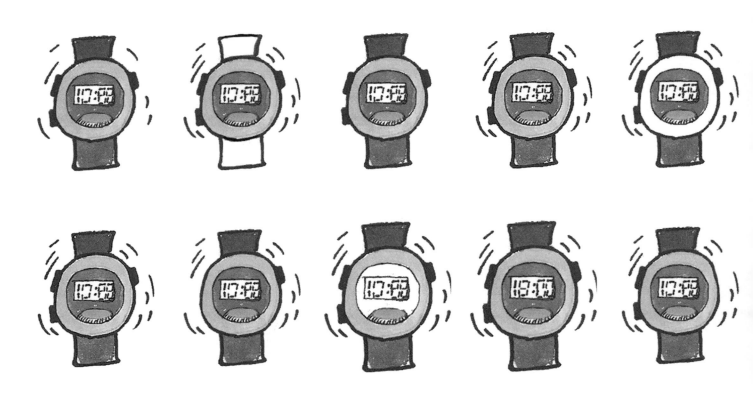

Find the Differences

Circle the 8 differences between the two drawings.

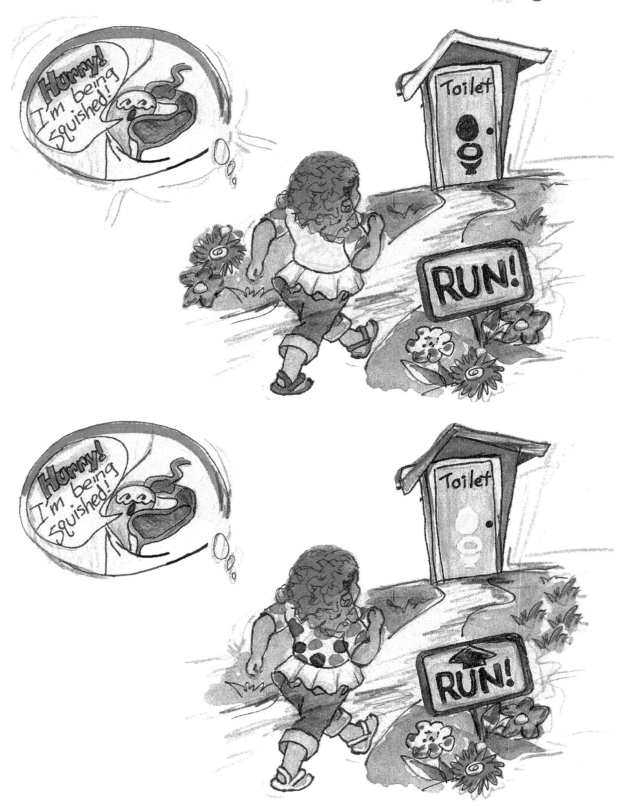

Did you know...?

When your rectum is stretched out by poop, it presses against the bladder, and this makes your bladder go nutty. That's why some constipated kids have to pee really badly or pee very often.

Here's how Dr. Pooper explains it in *Jane and the Giant Poop*.

"A bladder that's squished can get grouchy and mad, which makes children say, 'I have to pee REALLY bad!'"

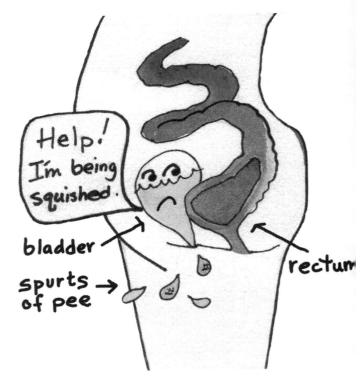

MAZE

Jane is at the toy store when she *really* has to pee. Help her find the toilet quickly!

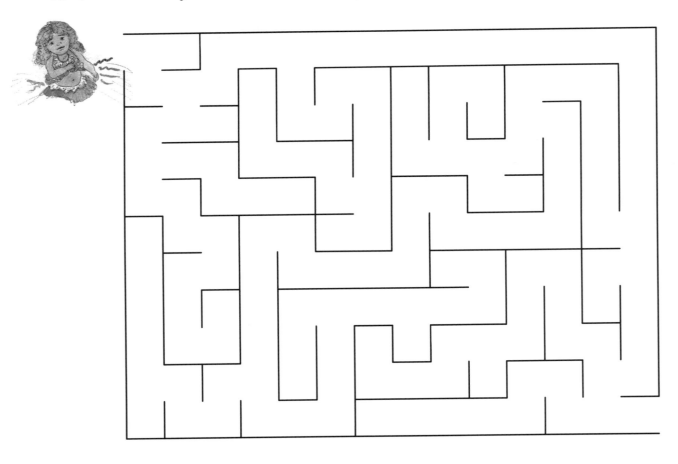

PART 4:
Accidents Are Never Your Fault!

Did you know...?

Children all over the world are constipated and have accidents! *Millions* of children! If you have accidents, you are definitely not the only one on in your neighborhood or at your school.

Color It!

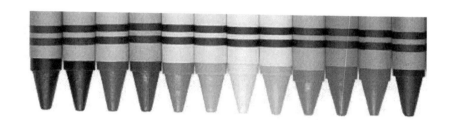

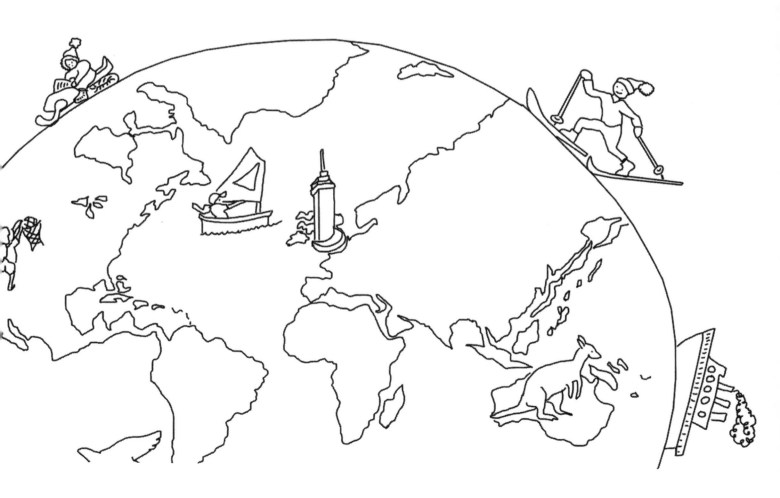

All Over the World

Beginner

Australia
Brazil
Canada
China

Egypt
France
Germany
Greece

India
Ireland
Israel
Italy

Japan
Kenya
Mexico
Norway

Russia
Spain
Sweden
Switzerland

```
          O U K E N Y A O
        G B N E I E C I T A L Y
        E W Q A M A I V O W J S A T
      Y N U R G W U U E G Y P T I A S
    S F H P K Y C G H V A B L K S S Y X
    Y M G B A U A E M P M E G N W P U I
  E S I M S T A N R S E S N R C E T W L U
  B P T O O B O A M T E X O E A D B D L V
  U A W T L N M D A W A Y I E A E L V Z J
  I I H V I P O A N U D L Q C B N B T Z A
  X N Z M E N D R Y C D Y F E O Y Z K K P
  L S F T A G M F W L O S I S R A E L W A
  C N E R R U S S I A Q P K V A H M X F N
  C Z B R A Z I L I L Y U F K A M N E W Z
  Z O E K N H E S W I T Z E R L A N D
  A P U A E C J C T U S F Z D M X M W
  G M Z M J E K H M B T C N D H Y
      A U S T R A L I A M U H Z Z
      T W I R E L A N D S H Z
        N I I N D I A H
```

Children in all these countries (and more!) have accidents. In the Beginner search, the words go across, downward, and diagonally. In the Advanced search, words also go backward.

Advanced

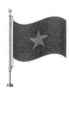

```
              E W M M Z R S R D M
              C O K T D W K O O O I Y N F
            P U A P F E D S C E W D U Z J L J N
          D H Y R Q N M D D W K S A A T R A Y I I
        M H W O D M D N A L E C I T D U H I S C W I
      L V C D K A H A A C M A N T E I V C E Z A C R P
    T C M E S R T L D Q X N H M X T K V B E Y R J U S
    O U X T K F R M T C N A R G E N T I N A E A Q H X H
  H W Q Z E J E F O W A S G K W T I Y A K K C G E G H F Q
  N I K C F H G X D B T N D T H A I L A N D R U L U Q J E
R M Q T V T X X Y G K I A Z G H K G N V W T T A I Y B R O I
P U C F E V D J R N K U J B A T S K U E B G Y T H I O Z K O
O I H N J D G Y A I R S M N N N B B N U C U U Q C P Q F J O
R G B B Z N K A G K F D E G A O I Y X Z W P J A A W S E R Y
T L T U G A D I N D E C E M W R H A O A R D W G T Y Z Q E E
U E E J K L E C U E W X Z Y I A K R B I Y L N W A E C B V K
G B J V H A A I H T I E I E A T T U V N Q I E V Z J M S T R
A W Z X O E I U X I E X L Z T A Q C C X S W V S N B Y A F U
L F M L N Z C N N U M E J F Q F G I A B Y E W Y Q E G L T
P F Y U D W D L E U Q I B M A Z O M C A V B V X O I Z B J A
  L M V U E O M N V M P O E S N N I B M K X G Y M H Q J D
    A F I R N N F K F W X S P U K R M V Q R U H F H U D M J
      U J A Q E L H W W F C V M F I T R M N L C A D D Q V
        T P S L S K U Q O O T G A Z S L C Q U U I V G W D S
          L E L I Z V A Y W A H S C O S K N P Y D J G V K
            M L A U F Z N W T Y C M O R O C C O O M M D
              X Q A T N A U X J N I E R N V K F O E N
                B Q O H O A I P O I H T E F N W K Y
                  N S J L S M V K X W B P A T
                  X W Y N A M I B I A
```

Argentina	Ethiopia	Morocco	Philippines	Tanzania
Belgium	Guatemala	Mozambique	Portugal	Thailand
Belize	Honduras	Namibia	Qatar	Turkey
Chile	Hungary	Netherlands	Singapore	United Kingdom
Denmark	Iceland	New Zealand	South Africa	Vietnam
Ecuador	Indonesia	Nicaragua	Taiwan	Zimbabwe

Did you know...?

When your rectum gets too stuffed with poop, it squishes the bladder, which can make the bladder hiccup! Pee can leak out before you can wake up or get to the bathroom.

Pee accidents are called **enuresis**.

WORDFINDER

How many words can you make out of **ENURESIS** (not including plurals)?

2-letter words: _____ _____ _____

3-letter words: _____ _____ _____ _____

_____ _____ _____ _____

_____ _____

4-letter words: _____ _____ _____

_____ _____ _____

_____ _____ _____

_____

5-letter words: _____ _____ _____

_____ _____ _____

_____ _____ _____

_____

6-letter words: _____ _____

7-letter words: _____ _____

WHICH TWO ARE IDENTICAL?

Circle the two squished bladders that are exactly the same.

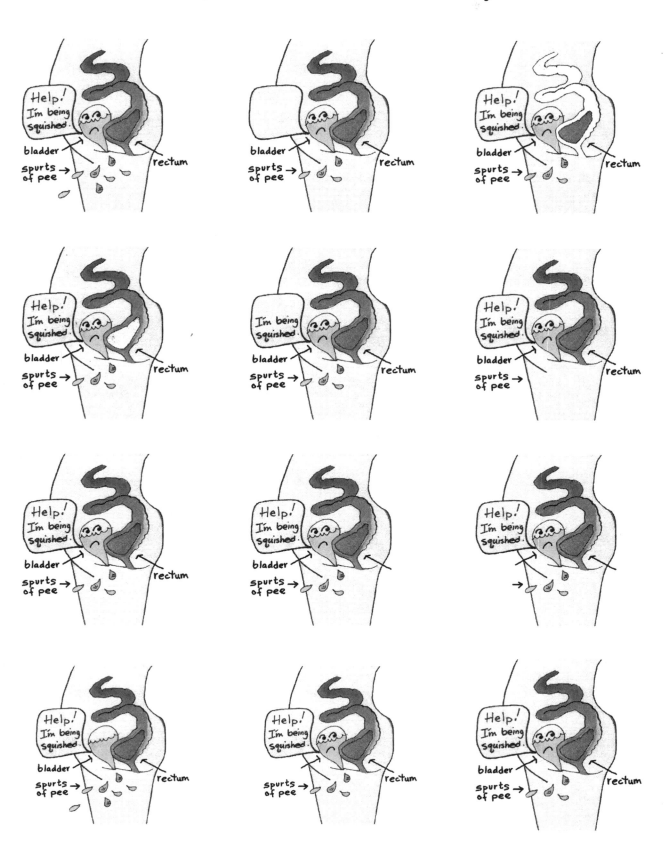

Did you know...?

When you clean out your rectum with enemas and mushy-poop medicine, your rectum will shrink back to regular size and stop squishing your bladder.

Sometimes fixing the problem can take a long time, so try to be patient!

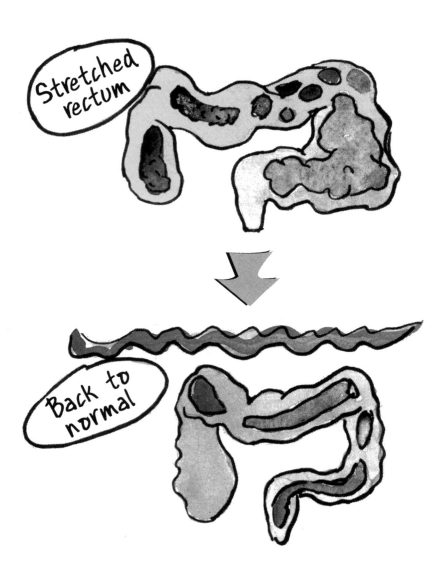

Stretched rectum

Back to normal

Rhyme It!

How many words can you rhyme with **SHRINK**?

_____   _____   _____   _____

_____   _____   _____   _____

_____   _____   _____   _____

_____   _____   _____   _____

_____

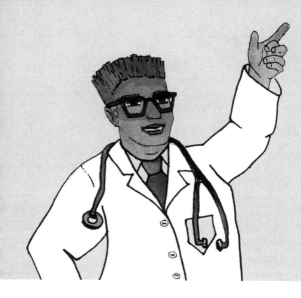

Dr. Pooper says...

**Accidents are like sneezes:
They come on very suddenly and
you just can't control them.**

**Sometimes adults wonder if kids wet
their bed or their pants on purpose.
But kids don't, of course!**

WHAT DID DR. POOPER SAY?

Cross out all the lower-case letters, g's and j's to find out what Dr. Pooper
says about accidents. Then copy the letters into the message below.

**A g C j g C I r D E m J N G T o S
j x w J m A g g o R J j p G E n l
G J N o p m O n j g J x q z e J T
i p G J y Y s a J O t m U G j x R
t o a J g F l m G A e U w L o T j**

——— —— —————— —————

—— ——————— ———

——— ——— ————

Did you know...?

Poop accidents are caused by constipation. When poop piles up in and stretches the rectum, the rectum becomes floppy, the way your t-shirt will get floppy if you stretch it over your knees.

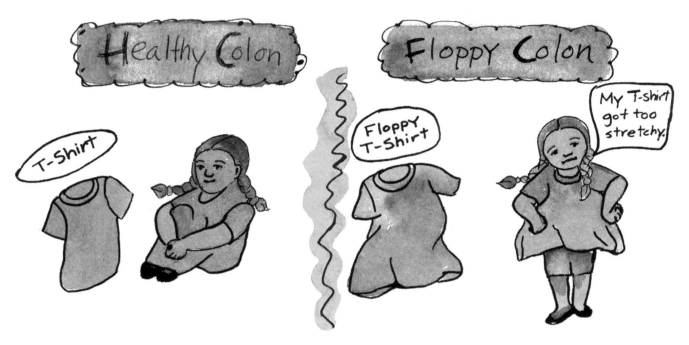

A floppy rectum can't hold in all your poop.
So, some of it just drops out your bottom.
You might not even feel the poop fall out.

Poop accidents are called **encopresis**.

Cleaning out your rectum every day with enemas will help it shrink back to regular size so the poop accidents will stop.

Rhyme It!

How many words can you rhyme with **FLOPPY**?

_____   _____   _____

WORDFINDER

How many words can you make out of **ENCOPRESIS** (not including plurals)?

2-letter words: _____ _____ _____ _____ _____ _____

3-letter words: _____ _____ _____ _____

_____ _____ _____ _____

_____ _____ _____ _____

_____ _____ _____ _____

4-letter words: _____ _____ _____

_____ _____ _____

_____ _____ _____

_____ _____ _____

_____ _____ _____

5-letter words: _____ _____ _____

_____ _____ _____

_____ _____ _____

_____ _____ _____

6-letter words: _____ _____

_____ _____

_____ _____

7-letter words: _____ _____

_____ _____

8-letter words: _____ _____

WHICH TWO ARE IDENTICAL?

Circle the two drawings that are exactly the same.

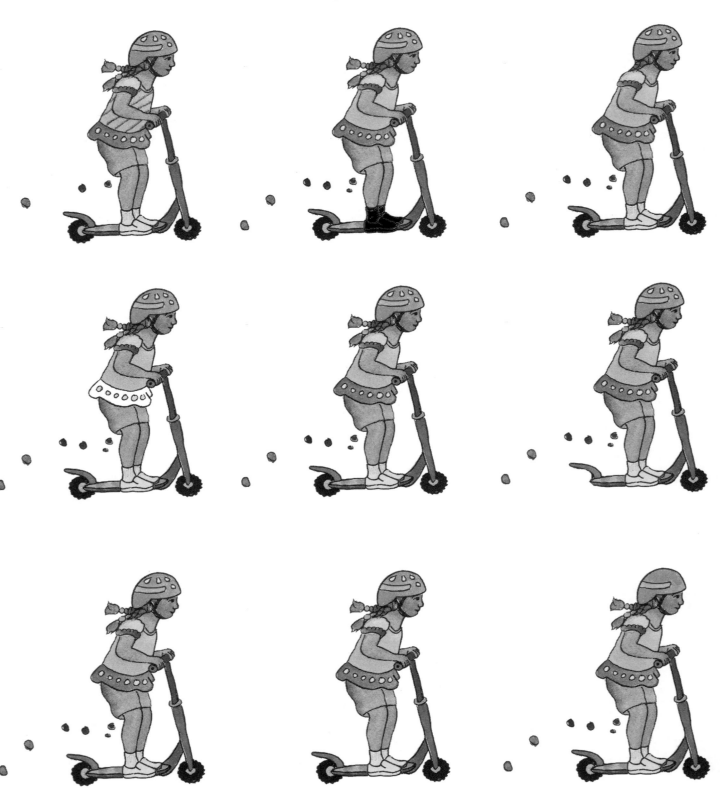

Dr. Pooper says...

It's really important to use the bathroom every two hours at school!

Holding in your pee or poop is not healthy for your bladder or rectum. Peeing often during the school day will help keep your bladder from going nutty and leaking at night.

If your teacher has a rule against using the bathroom during class time, tell a parent, so your mom or dad can talk to your teacher. Your teacher will understand!

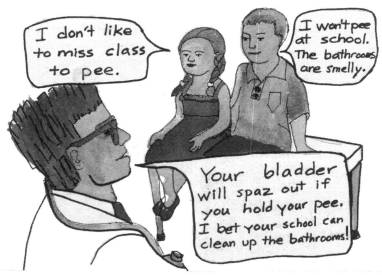

Jane and her teacher have a secret code for communicating during class. Using Morse Code, she signals this secret message during class.

DECODE THE MESSAGE

I · ·
D — · ·
P · — — ·
N — ·
T —
E ·
O — — —

· · / — · / · / · / — · · / — / — — — / · — — · / · / · /

The slash mark (/) in the message is the space between the letters.

MAZE

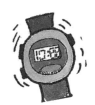

Zoe's potty watch just vibrated during recess!
Help her get to the bathroom right right away.

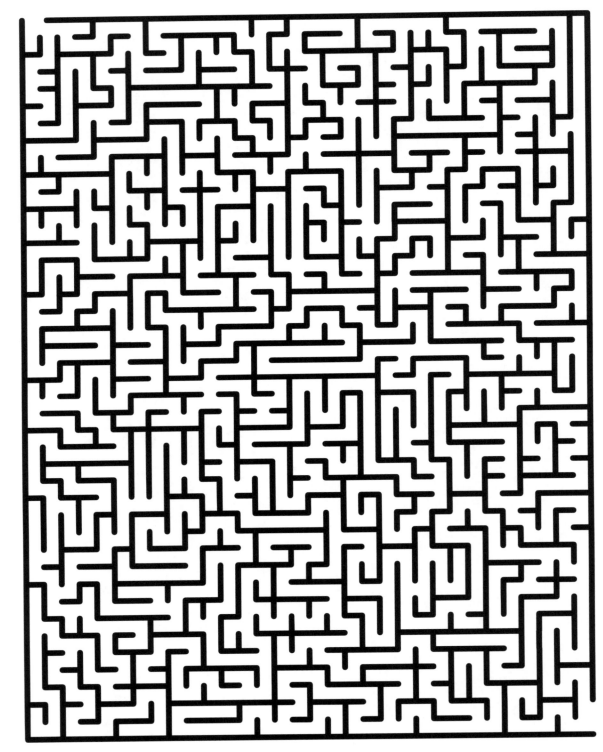

WORDFINDER

How many words can you make out of **BATHROOM**?

2-letter words: _____ _____ _____ _____ _____

_____ _____

3-letter words: _____ _____ _____ _____

_____ _____ _____ _____

_____ _____ _____ _____

_____ _____ _____ _____

_____ _____ _____ _____

_____

4-letter words: _____ _____ _____

_____ _____ _____

_____ _____ _____

_____ _____ _____

_____ _____ _____

_____ _____ _____

_____

5-letter words: _____ _____ _____

_____ _____ _____

_____ _____

Find the Mystery Words

Unscramble these bathroom words. Then, transfer the shaded letters to spell an important message about using the bathroom!

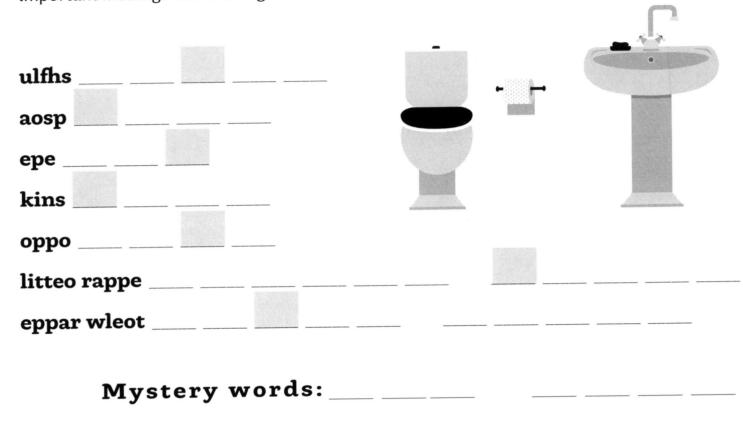

ulfhs _____ _____ _____ _____ _____

aosp _____ _____ _____ _____

epe _____ _____ _____

kins _____ _____ _____ _____

oppo _____ _____ _____ _____

litteo rappe _____ _____ _____ _____ _____ _____ _____ _____ _____ _____ _____

eppar wleot _____ _____ _____ _____ _____ _____ _____ _____ _____ _____ _____

Mystery words: _____ _____ _____ _____ _____ _____ _____

Rhyme It!

How many words can you rhyme with **SINK**?

_____ _____ _____ _____

_____ _____ _____ _____

_____ _____ _____ _____

Dr. Pooper says...

Drinking lots of water keeps your bladder healthy and helps keep your poop mushy! Keep a water bottle on your desk at school, and drink from it often.

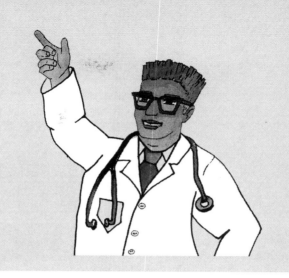

WHICH TWO ARE IDENTICAL?

Zack and Zoe's class has 20 students. But only Zack and Zoe have the same exact water bottle. Can you find their bottles?

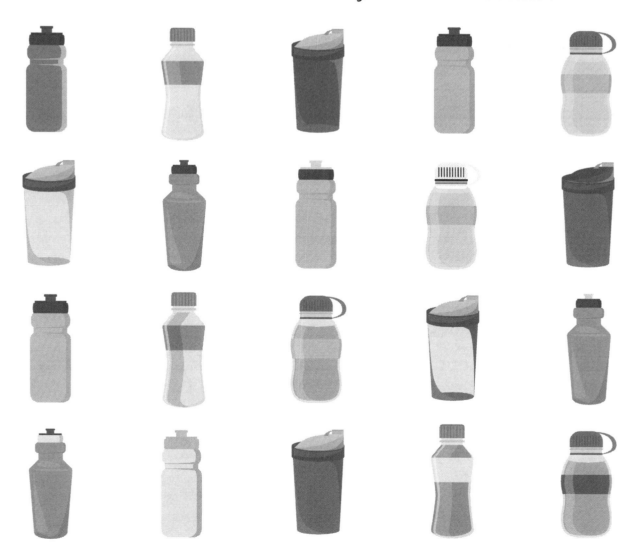

Find the Differences

Circle the 8 differences between these two drawings.

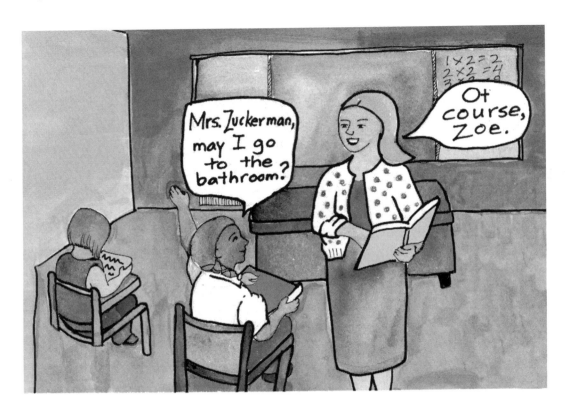

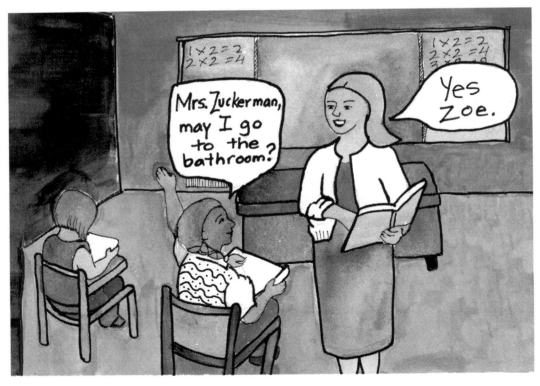

PART 6:
Eating for Mushy Poop

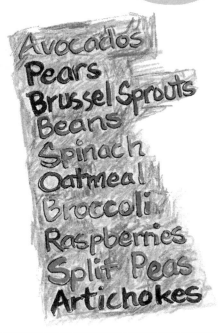

Avocados
Pears
Brussel Sprouts
Beans
Spinach
Oatmeal
Broccoli
Raspberries
Split Peas
Artichokes

Did you know...?

Eating lots of fruits and veggies helps keep your poop soft, so pooping doesn't hurt. Eat at least one fruit or vegetable with every meal. Better yet, eat two!

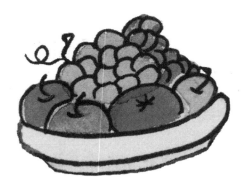

WORD SCRAMBLE

These five foods are technically fruits, but most people mistake them for vegetables. Can you unscramble them?

rumccueb

doovcaa

mootta

voile

kpmupni

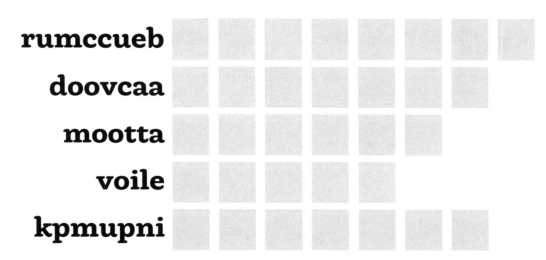

Word Search: *A Fruitful Search*

How many fruits can you find? The words go across, downward, and diagonally.

Apple	Cherry	Guava	Orange	Pomegranate
Apricot	Cranberry	Honeydew	Papaya	Raspberry
Banana	Date	Kiwi	Peach	Starfruit
Blackberry	Fig	Lemon	Pear	Strawberry
Blueberry	Grapefruit	Mango	Pineapple	Tangerine
Cantaloupe	Grapes	Nectarine	Plum	Watermelon

```
                              E
                           J  B  M
                        L  Z  Z  O  K
                           E  T  M  I  A
                           M  A  I  Y  R
                           O  N  S  B
         L  D  K  P  R  Q     Q  U  N  G  O  Z     A  Q  N  L  P
      C  H  O  N  E  Y  D  E  W  X  I  X  N  E  N  E  C  T  A  R  I  N  E  J
      O  A  L  O  T  P  L  U  M  Z  B  D  T  F  O  R  A  N  G  E  A  D  W  U  Q  M
      B  N  Z  D  F  V  U  Y  G  A  C  T  O  A  R  O  I  X  A  O  F  E  A  O  C  M  O
   B  N  T  I  M  B  B  L  A  C  K  B  E  R  R  Y  B  S  N  D  L  Q  Q  T  M  O  C  A
   J  J  A  S  D  C  N  C  S  D  H  K  M  C  H  E  R  R  Y  E  P  V  B  E  K  J  F  K
   B  P  L  Y  L  R  M  Y  L  I  X  Z  I  K  E  S  L  Z  Y  D  R  I  E  R  L  Z  J  I  U
B  B  A  O  N  O  A  N  R  Z  W  P  N  F  F  I  G  Y  G  K  A  H  U  N  M  H  X  I  W  O
L  S  H  U  A  Y  N  M  M  Z  G  O  M  C  Z  L  T  N  R  D  T  N  Q  W  E  N  A  P  I  V
U  F  A  P  O  U  B  X  D  M  G  M  O  U  R  O  A  O  A  B  E  A  I  C  L  A  F  A  F  F
E  V  F  E  O  E  E  G  R  A  G  E  U  N  B  D  G  I  P  G  J  B  L  M  O  E  P  Q  A  Z
B  Y  Q  A  R  T  R  D  W  N  H  G  P  J  R  O  T  M  E  Z  G  G  I  X  N  E  A  P  Z  M
E  H  X  M  V  G  R  G  T  G  M  R  T  A  F  J  Y  H  F  P  Q  U  D  M  M  T  R  X  L  N
R  G  A  Z  I  J  Y  R  E  O  Z  A  E  A  P  M  L  U  R  T  T  A  K  R  C  R  Q  H  H  E
R  X  M  P  K  I  R  A  D  S  D  N  R  S  T  A  Y  R  U  F  N  V  C  E  P  T  Y  S  M  A
Y  D  M  F  R  E  E  P  A  E  H  A  Q  T  T  Q  Y  B  I  W  Y  A  W  E  B  S  E  D  I
N  N  J  V  I  G  E  R  F  H  T  D  A  A  J  V  A  T  S  I  T  K  B  P  E  A  C  H
A  W  T  V  F  C  S  Y  U  K  E  A  R  N  K  S  Z  J  D  F  F  F  A  P  P  L  E  T
   Z  X  I  D  O  O  A  M  N  H  P  F  B  A  N  A  N  A  D  S  H  D  Y  N  V  K
      Y  F  F  A  K  T  U  B  O  E  R  Z  N  N  S  M  F  D  F  G  H  R  O  W
         E  P  H  Q  Y  J  P  U  A  U  D  T  S  T  R  A  W  B  E  R  R  Y
            N  N  Y  G  A  G  W  R  I  R  A  S  P  B  E  R  R  Y  W  Q
               F  T  Q  T  B  S  W  C  D
               L  K  S  V  Y  U  F
```

WHICH TWO ARE IDENTICAL?

Jane's favorite fruit is watermelon.
Which two watermelons are identical?

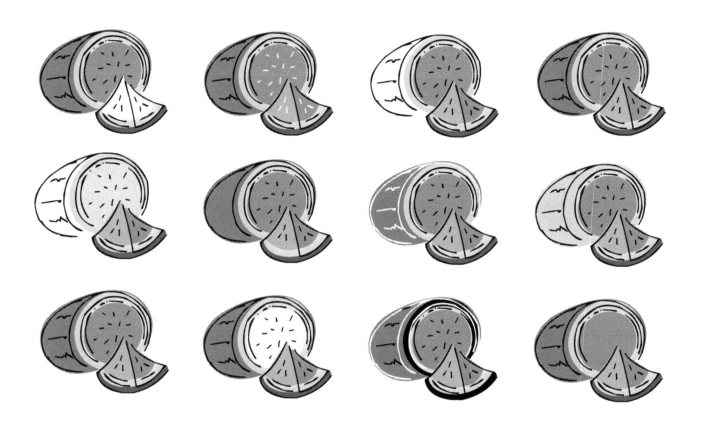

Dr. Pooper
wants to know:

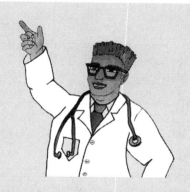

What are your 3 favorite fruits?

1. _____

2. _____

3. _____

What are your 3 favorite vegetables?

1. _____

2. _____

3. _____

How many words can you make out of **SPINACH** (not including plurals)?

2-letter words: _____ _____ _____ _____ _____ _____ _____

_____

3-letter words: _____ _____ _____ _____

_____ _____ _____ _____

_____ _____ _____ _____

4-letter words: _____ _____ _____

_____ _____ _____

_____ _____ _____

_____ _____ _____

_____

5-letter words: _____ _____ _____

_____

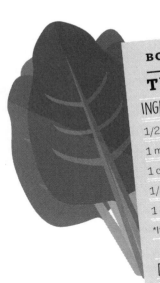

BONUS RECIPE: Here's the recipe for a delicious green smoothie! Make it at home!

The Incredible Hulk Smoothie – Makes two 1-cup smoothies

INGREDIENT LIST:

1/2 cup cold water

1 medium banana, frozen and cut or broken into a few pieces

1 cup pineapple (canned)*

1/4 cup pineapple juice (use the juice from the canned pineapple)

1 cup packed fresh baby spinach

*If using fresh pineapple, omit pineapple juice, increase water to 3/4 cup, and add a teaspoon of honey

DIRECTIONS:

Put all ingredients in a high-powered blender in the order listed.

Blend until smooth and serve immediately.

Reprinted with permission from RealMomNutrition.com

CROSSWORD

Go Green!

All the words below are green vegetables. Use the clues to fill in the blanks.

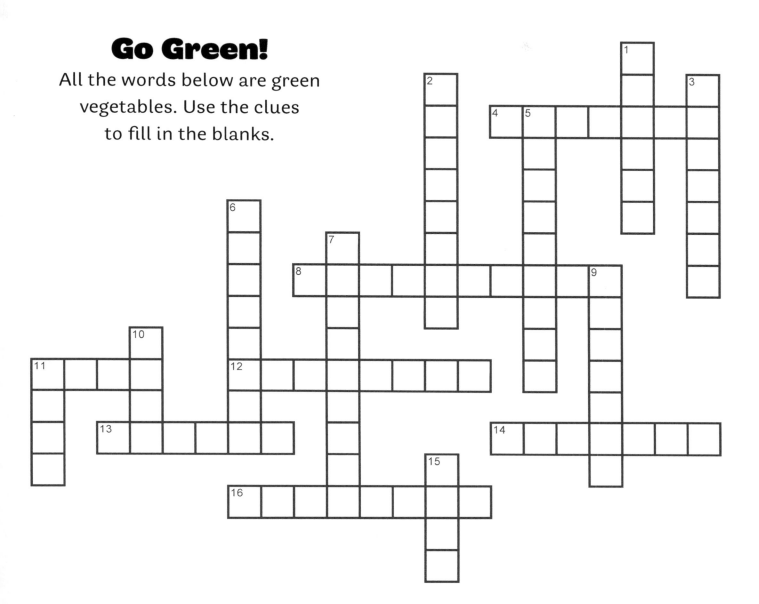

Across:

4 Comes in green and purple

8 AKA string beans

11 Hairy on the outside, sweet on the inside

12 A cousin of cauliflower

13 Use it to make ants on a log

14 Mash it into "guac"

16 A cousin of cantaloupe

Down:

1 Grown on a vine

2 A summer squash

3 Part of a BLT

5 Long and skinny and makes your pee stink!

6 Has a waxy peel

7 Its heart is delicious

9 Brighten up your smoothie with a bunch of this

10 It's "key" to a tart pie

11 Drizzle with oil and roast to make yummy chips!

15 Find them in a pod

MAZE

Zack and his mom are at the grocery store shopping for fruit.
Help them find their way through the produce section!

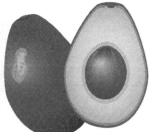

RECIPES

Here are two yummy recipes you can make with fruit!

Creamy Chocolate Banana Pudding - Makes about eight 1/2-cup servings

INGREDIENT LIST:

2 ripe avocados

4 ripe bananas, peeled

1/2 cup plus 3 tablespoons unsweetened cocoa powder

1/2 cup unsweetened coconut milk or cow's milk

1-1/2 teaspoons pure vanilla extract

4 to 5 tablespoons pure maple syrup

DIRECTIONS:

Scoop out the flesh of the avocado and place in a food processor or high-speed blender.

Add remaining ingredients.

Process until creamy, stopping to scrape down the sides. Add additional maple syrup to taste.

Serve immediately or store in air-tight container in refrigerator.

Reprinted with permission from School-Bites.com

Fluffy Blueberry Pancakes - Makes about 12 pancakes

INGREDIENT LIST:

1 large egg

1 cup white whole wheat flour

1 cup milk

1 tablespoon honey

1 tablespoon canola oil

3 tablespoons ground flaxseed

2 teaspoons baking powder

1/2 teaspoon vanilla

1/8 teaspoon salt

1 cup frozen blueberries

1/2 tablespoon butter, melted

DIRECTIONS:

Beat egg until light and fluffy. Add flour and remaining ingredients (through salt) and stir just until combined. Fold frozen blueberries into batter.

While batter rests, preheat skillet. Brush melted butter onto surface. When skillet sizzles, drop batter on using a quarter-cup measure. When surface bubbles and bottom is brown, flip pancakes. Repeat until batter is done.

Reprinted with permission from RealMomNutrition.com

Did you know...?

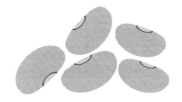

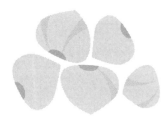

Beans are loaded with fiber, which helps water stay in your poop. That makes your poop softer, so you can poop more easily!

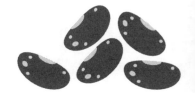

WORDFINDER

Garbanzo beans are also called chickpeas and are great for making yummy snacks, like hummus and cinnamon-roasted chickpeas.

How many words can you find in **GARBANZO**?

2-letter words: _____   _____   _____   _____

3-letter words: _____   _____   _____   _____

_____   _____   _____   _____

_____   _____   _____   _____

_____   _____   _____   _____

_____   _____

4-letter words: _____   _____   _____

_____   _____   _____

_____   _____   _____

5-letter words: _____   _____

Word Search: *Beans, Beans, Beans!*

Find all these beans! The words go across, downward, and diagonally.

Adzuki
Black
Blackeyedpeas
Cannellini

Fava
Garbanzo
Greatnorthern
Kidney

Lentils
Lima
Mung
Navy

Pinto
Red
Soybean
Splitpeas

```
S  P  L  I  T  P  E  A  S  M  K  K  A  P  D
P  P  C  D  V  N  B  V  M  N  M  F  A  V  A
K  W  J  B  L  E  K  I  D  N  E  Y  V  D  A
G  R  E  A  T  N  O  R  T  H  E  R  N  X  D
S  I  Z  B  G  U  W  O  X  N  V  Q  K  W  Z
C  M  P  L  N  I  H  Q  W  N  D  E  S  C  U
A  V  M  A  D  P  I  N  T  O  I  R  O  K  K
N  Z  T  C  X  R  U  O  N  O  P  E  Y  G  I
N  H  C  K  K  U  A  N  A  V  Y  D  B  U  D
E  S  V  D  Q  W  G  X  C  Z  P  R  E  B  J
L  B  L  A  C  K  E  Y  E  D  P  E  A  S  C
L  Z  M  D  H  S  I  G  A  R  B  A  N  Z  O
I  Z  U  K  G  Y  D  J  Y  Z  T  S  A  I  N
N  V  N  C  L  I  M  A  C  X  X  O  S  X  D
I  J  G  R  L  M  L  E  N  T  I  L  S  P  I
```

RECIPES

Here are two great recipes you can make with beans.

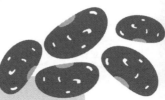

Very Lemony Homemade Hummus

INGREDIENT LIST:

2 (15-ounce cans) chickpeas (drain and reserve the liquid)

Juice of 3 lemons

1 teaspoon salt

Ground pepper to taste

1 clove chopped garlic (or 1/2 tsp. jarred minced garlic)

3 tablespoons tahini paste (found in "ethnic foods" section)

1/4 cup olive oil

DIRECTIONS:

Place beans, lemon juice, salt, pepper, garlic, and tahini in blender or food processor. As you blend, drizzle in olive oil.

Scrape side and continue to blend, drizzling in reserved liquid from beans until you get the consistency you want.

Store in the refrigerator in an air-tight container.

Reprinted with permission from RealMomNutrition.com

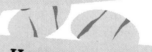

Hearty Beans and Greens Soup - Serves 6 to 8

INGREDIENT LIST:

2 tablespoons olive oil

1 medium yellow onion, chopped

2 ribs celery, thinly sliced

4 cloves garlic, finely chopped

1 teaspoon kosher salt

8 cups low-sodium chicken broth

1 pound Yukon Gold or russet potatoes (2 medium), cut into 1/2-inch pieces

1 bunch kale, stemmed and torn into small pieces

1 tablespoon chopped fresh rosemary

2 (15.5-ounce) cans cannellini beans, rinsed and drained

1/4 cup (1 ounce) grated Parmesan cheese

1/2 teaspoon black pepper

DIRECTIONS:

Heat oil in a large pot over medium-high heat. Add onion, celery, garlic, and 1/2 teaspoon salt and cook, stirring often, until softened, about 10 minutes.

Add chicken broth and bring to a boil. Add potatoes, kale, rosemary, and the remaining 1/2 teaspoon salt and simmer until the vegetables are tender, about 15 minutes. Stir in beans, Parmesan, and pepper.

Simmer to heat through.

Refrigerate in an airtight container for up to 4 days or freeze for up to 2 months.

Reprinted with permission from The Good Neighbor Cookbook

PART 7:
Moving Your Body

Did you know...?

Moving your body helps keep
your poop moving through
your colon! It's important to
be active every day.

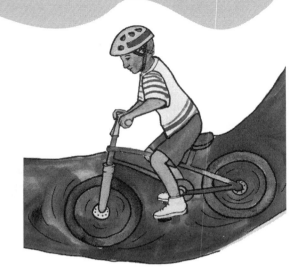

MAZE

Zack loves to ride his bike through the park.
Help him find his way back home.

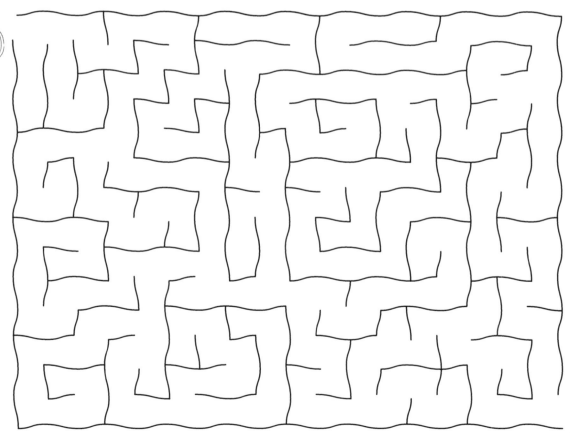

Word Search: *Get Moving!*

Sports keep poop moving through your colon!
The words go across, downward, and diagonally.

baseball
basketball
bicycling
dance

football
gymnastics
hiking
hockey

jumping rope
kickball
lacrosse
running

skateboarding
skiing
softball
swimming

tennis
volleyball
walking
yoga

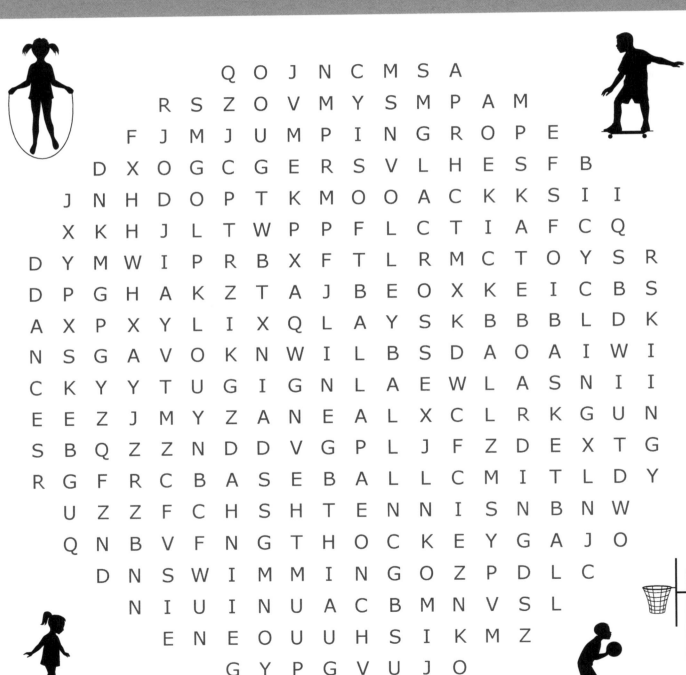

```
      Q O J N C M S A
      R S Z O V M Y S M P A M
      F J M J U M P I N G R O P E
    D X O G C G E R S V L H E S F B
  J N H D O P T K M O O A C K K S I I
  X K H J L T W P P F L C T I A F C Q
D Y M W I P R B X F T L R M C T O Y S R
D P G H A K Z T A J B E O X K E I C B S
A X P X Y L I X Q L A Y S K B B B L D K
N S G A V O K N W I L B S D A O A I W I
C K Y Y T U G I G N L A E W L A S N I I
E E Z J M Y Z A N E A L X C L R K G U N
S B Q Z Z N D D V G P L J F Z D E X T G
R G F R C B A S E B A L L C M I T L D Y
U Z Z F C H S T E N N I S N B N W
Q N B V F N G T H O C K E Y G A J O
  D N S W I M M I N G O Z P D L C
    N I U I N U A C B M N V S L
    E N E O U U H S I K M Z
      G Y P G V U J O
```

WHICH TWO ARE IDENTICAL?

Circle the two pictures of Zoe that are exactly alike.

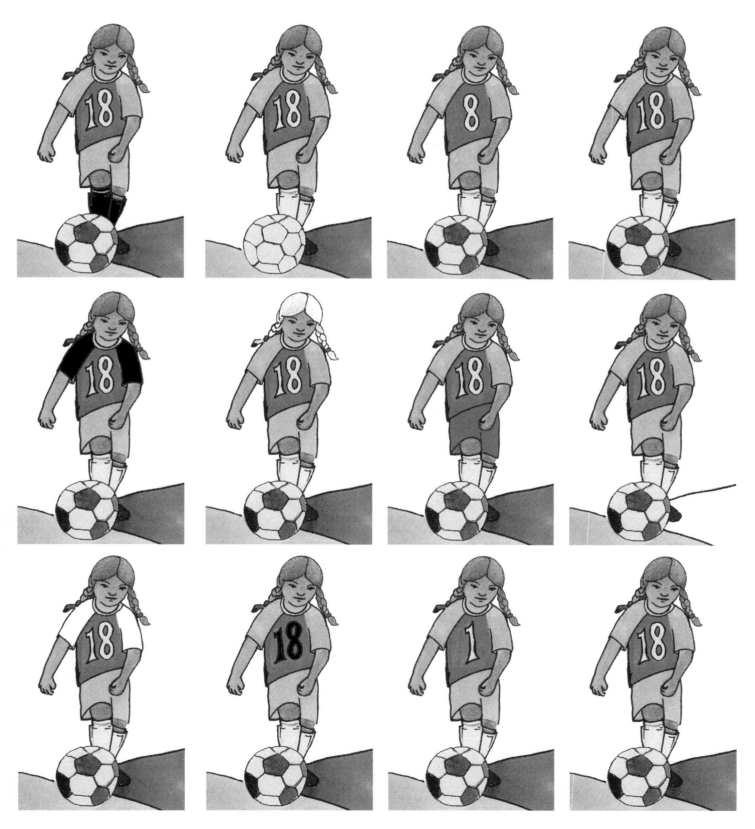

Learn to Draw

Follow these 4 steps to draw a dog!

How to Draw a Dog

#1

a. sketch box around the dog
b. make dash lines in a t-shape ---|---

#2

a. make your own box
b. add the t-shape ---|---

#3

a. look at drawing #1 and fill in each of the four squares

#4

a. erase the extra lines

Now, draw your own dog.

Draw Your Own Dog

Start with this example →

Now, make your own drawing

MAZE

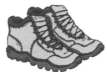

Jane loves to hike with her dad.
Help them find their way to the lake.

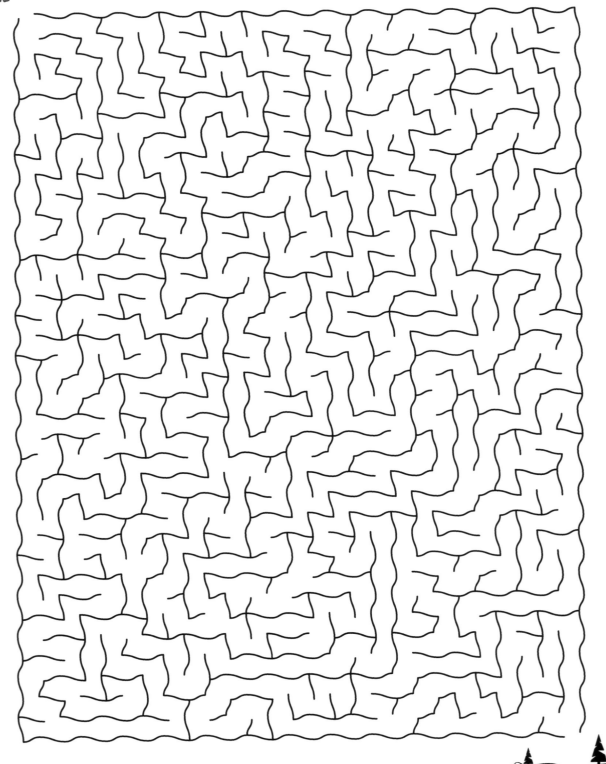

UNCOVER A MESSAGE

Cross out all the capital letters, m's and w's to find out Dr. Pooper's three favorite activities. Then copy the letters into the message below.

**W T r m u w n A n S i P n m g w
b Y a s C k m e P t m b E a l M l
m W s D o P m c T c m w e M r**

_____

_____

_____

Jane loves to jump rope and do yoga.
Zoe loves to play soccer and ride her scooter.
Zack loves to ride his bike and run.

What are your three favorite activities?

1. _____

2. _____

3. _____

Rhyme It!

How many words can you rhyme with **DANCE**?

_____   _____   _____

_____   _____   _____

How many words can you rhyme with **JUMP**?

_____   _____   _____

_____   _____   _____

WORDFINDER

How many words can you find in **SCOOTER** (not including plurals)?

2-letter words: _____   _____   _____

3-letter words: _____   _____   _____   _____

_____   _____   _____

4-letter words: _____   _____   _____

_____   _____   _____

_____   _____   _____

_____   _____

5-letter words: _____   _____   _____

_____   _____   _____

6-letter words: _____   _____

_____

How many words can you find in **KICKBALL**?

3-letter words: _____   _____   _____   _____

_____   _____   _____

4-letter words: _____   _____   _____

_____   _____   _____

_____   _____   _____

5-letter words: _____   _____

PART 8:
Charting Your Poop

WEEK 1 Color Your Poop

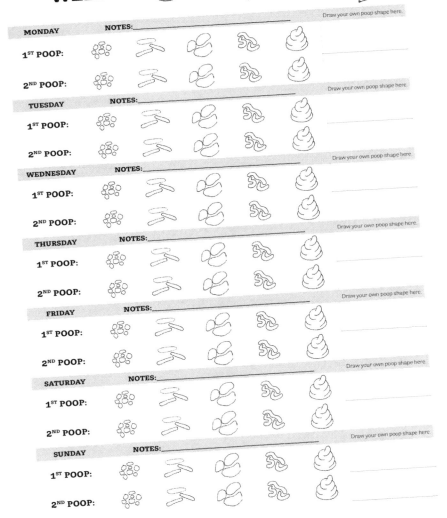

Did you know...?

It's important to poop every single day! Keep track of what your poop looks like using these charts.

Each time you poop, look at what you made in the toilet (yes, it's kind of gross!) and notice the shape. Then, color in the shape that looks the most like your poop.
Or, draw your own!

Try it for a week!

WEEK 1 Color Your Poop

MONDAY	NOTES:_____	Draw your own poop shape here.
1ST POOP:		
2ND POOP:		

TUESDAY	NOTES:_____	Draw your own poop shape here.
1ST POOP:		
2ND POOP:		

WEDNESDAY	NOTES:_____	Draw your own poop shape here.
1ST POOP:		
2ND POOP:		

THURSDAY	NOTES:_____	Draw your own poop shape here.
1ST POOP:		
2ND POOP:		

FRIDAY	NOTES:_____	Draw your own poop shape here.
1ST POOP:		
2ND POOP:		

SATURDAY	NOTES:_____	Draw your own poop shape here.
1ST POOP:		
2ND POOP:		

SUNDAY	NOTES:_____	Draw your own poop shape here.
1ST POOP:		
2ND POOP:		

WEEK 2

Color Your Poop

| MONDAY | NOTES: _____ | Draw your own poop shape here. |

1ST POOP:

2ND POOP:

| TUESDAY | NOTES: _____ | Draw your own poop shape here. |

1ST POOP:

2ND POOP:

| WEDNESDAY | NOTES: _____ | Draw your own poop shape here. |

1ST POOP:

2ND POOP:

| THURSDAY | NOTES: _____ | Draw your own poop shape here. |

1ST POOP:

2ND POOP:

| FRIDAY | NOTES: _____ | Draw your own poop shape here. |

1ST POOP:

2ND POOP:

| SATURDAY | NOTES: _____ | Draw your own poop shape here. |

1ST POOP:

2ND POOP:

| SUNDAY | NOTES: _____ | Draw your own poop shape here. |

1ST POOP:

2ND POOP:

WEEK 3 — Color Your Poop

| MONDAY | NOTES:_____ | Draw your own poop shape here. |

1ST POOP:

2ND POOP:

| TUESDAY | NOTES:_____ | Draw your own poop shape here. |

1ST POOP:

2ND POOP:

| WEDNESDAY | NOTES:_____ | Draw your own poop shape here. |

1ST POOP:

2ND POOP:

| THURSDAY | NOTES:_____ | Draw your own poop shape here. |

1ST POOP:

2ND POOP:

| FRIDAY | NOTES:_____ | Draw your own poop shape here. |

1ST POOP:

2ND POOP:

| SATURDAY | NOTES:_____ | Draw your own poop shape here. |

1ST POOP:

2ND POOP:

| SUNDAY | NOTES:_____ | Draw your own poop shape here. |

1ST POOP:

2ND POOP:

WEEK 4 Color Your Poop

MONDAY	NOTES:_____	Draw your own poop shape here.
1ST POOP:		
2ND POOP:		

TUESDAY	NOTES:_____	Draw your own poop shape here.
1ST POOP:		
2ND POOP:		

WEDNESDAY	NOTES:_____	Draw your own poop shape here.
1ST POOP:		
2ND POOP:		

THURSDAY	NOTES:_____	Draw your own poop shape here.
1ST POOP:		
2ND POOP:		

FRIDAY	NOTES:_____	Draw your own poop shape here.
1ST POOP:		
2ND POOP:		

SATURDAY	NOTES:_____	Draw your own poop shape here.
1ST POOP:		
2ND POOP:		

SUNDAY	NOTES:_____	Draw your own poop shape here.
1ST POOP:		
2ND POOP:		

WEEK 5 Color Your Poop

MONDAY	NOTES:_____	Draw your own poop shape here.
1ST POOP:		
2ND POOP:		

TUESDAY	NOTES:_____	Draw your own poop shape here.
1ST POOP:		
2ND POOP:		

WEDNESDAY	NOTES:_____	Draw your own poop shape here.
1ST POOP:		
2ND POOP:		

THURSDAY	NOTES:_____	Draw your own poop shape here.
1ST POOP:		
2ND POOP:		

FRIDAY	NOTES:_____	Draw your own poop shape here.
1ST POOP:		
2ND POOP:		

SATURDAY	NOTES:_____	Draw your own poop shape here.
1ST POOP:		
2ND POOP:		

SUNDAY	NOTES:_____	Draw your own poop shape here.
1ST POOP:		
2ND POOP:		

WEEK 6   *Color Your Poop*

MONDAY   NOTES:_____   Draw your own poop shape here.

1ST POOP:

2ND POOP:

TUESDAY   NOTES:_____   Draw your own poop shape here.

1ST POOP:

2ND POOP:

WEDNESDAY   NOTES:_____   Draw your own poop shape here.

1ST POOP:

2ND POOP:

THURSDAY   NOTES:_____   Draw your own poop shape here.

1ST POOP:

2ND POOP:

FRIDAY   NOTES:_____   Draw your own poop shape here.

1ST POOP:

2ND POOP:

SATURDAY   NOTES:_____   Draw your own poop shape here.

1ST POOP:

2ND POOP:

SUNDAY   NOTES:_____   Draw your own poop shape here.

1ST POOP:

2ND POOP:

WEEK 7 Color Your Poop

MONDAY	NOTES:_____					Draw your own poop shape here.
1ST POOP:						
2ND POOP:						

TUESDAY	NOTES:_____					Draw your own poop shape here.
1ST POOP:						
2ND POOP:						

WEDNESDAY	NOTES:_____					Draw your own poop shape here.
1ST POOP:						
2ND POOP:						

THURSDAY	NOTES:_____					Draw your own poop shape here.
1ST POOP:						
2ND POOP:						

FRIDAY	NOTES:_____					Draw your own poop shape here.
1ST POOP:						
2ND POOP:						

SATURDAY	NOTES:_____					Draw your own poop shape here.
1ST POOP:						
2ND POOP:						

SUNDAY	NOTES:_____					Draw your own poop shape here.
1ST POOP:						
2ND POOP:						

WEEK 8 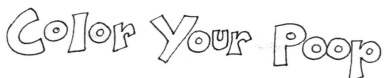 Color Your Poop

MONDAY   NOTES:_____   Draw your own poop shape here.

1ST POOP:

2ND POOP:

TUESDAY   NOTES:_____   Draw your own poop shape here.

1ST POOP:

2ND POOP:

WEDNESDAY   NOTES:_____   Draw your own poop shape here.

1ST POOP:

2ND POOP:

THURSDAY   NOTES:_____   Draw your own poop shape here.

1ST POOP:

2ND POOP:

FRIDAY   NOTES:_____   Draw your own poop shape here.

1ST POOP:

2ND POOP:

SATURDAY   NOTES:_____   Draw your own poop shape here.

1ST POOP:

2ND POOP:

SUNDAY   NOTES:_____   Draw your own poop shape here.

1ST POOP:

2ND POOP:

Part 9:
Answers

page 3

WORDFINDER:
Possible words in PUDDING:
2-letter words: up, in
3-letter words: nip, pig, pin, pug, pun, did, gnu, dig, din, dip, dud, dug, gun, gin

page 8

FLUSH:
Possible rhymes: blush, brush, crush, gush, hush, lush, mush, plush, rush, slush

CLOG:
Possible rhymes: blog, bog, dog, flog, fog, frog, hog, jog, log, slog, smog

page 10

MYSTERY WORDS:
Mushy poop
UNSCRAMBLED WORDS:
hummus, frozen yogurt, snake, milkshake, cow patty, pudding, log, blobs, pellets

WORDFINDER:
Possible words in SAUSAGE:
2-letter words: us, as
3-letter words: sea, sue, use, age, gas, sag
4-letter words: sags, uses, sage, seas, ages, sues
5-letter words: gases, sagas, sages, usage, guess

page 4

WORD SEARCH:
SHAPES OF POOP

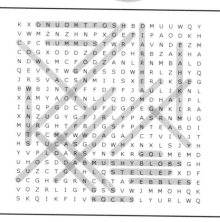

page 9

MATCH THE SHADOW

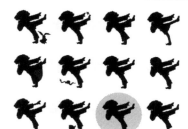

page 14

FIND THE DIFFERENCES:

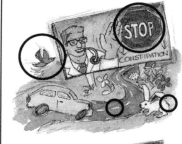
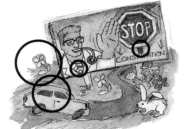

page 15

MAZE:

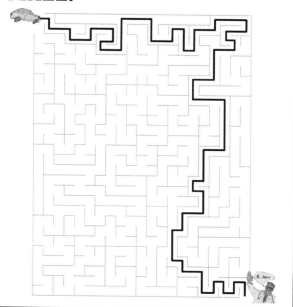

page 16

DECODE THE MESSAGE:
Poop every day

RHYME IT!
POOP
Possible rhymes: coop, coupe, croup, droop, dupe, goop, group, hoop, loop, scoop, snoop, soup, stoop, swoop, troop, troupe, whoop
WIPE
Possible rhymes: gripe, hype, pipe, stripe, swipe, type

page 17

WHICH IS DIFFERENT?

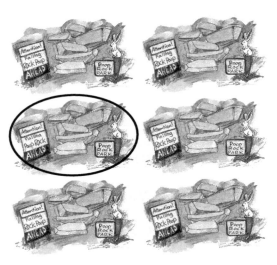

page 18

WHICH TWO ARE IDENTICAL?:

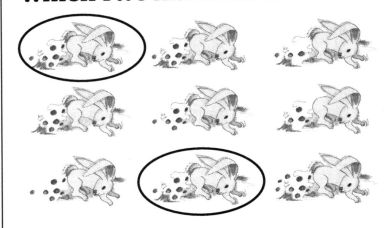

WHAT DID JANE SAY?:
Hard as a rock

page 19

WORDFINDER: Possible words in MILKSHAKES:
2-letter words: ma, as, am, is, me, hi, he
3-letter words: sea, ski, she, ail, has, hem, him, his, ilk, ham, aim, ale, ash, ask, elk, elm, lie
4-letter words: lake, meal, sake, mesh, sale, lame, lima, mail, lies, like, make, male, mask, mash, lash, sale, leak, mile, milk, elms, hail, hale, elks, ails, aims, slim, slam, alms, skim, silk, sham, slam, kale, seal, seam, lime, heal, same, helm, hike, isle
5-letter words: heals, shale, leash, shame, likes, hails, shake, lakes, hikes, leaks, aisle, makes, mails, males, meals, alike, miles, milks, limes, smile, slime

page 20

RHYME IT! SPLASH
Possible rhymes: ash, bash, brash, cash, clash, crash, dash, flash, gash, gnash, hash, mash, rash, sash, slash, smash, stash, thrash, trash

page 21

WORDFINDER:

Possible words in PLUNGER:

3-letter words: pun, gun, urn, run, gel, gnu, leg, lug, peg, pen, per, pug

4-letter words: lung, lure, pure, luge, plug, urge, rung, gulp, glue, rule

5-letter words: gruel, purge, prune, lunge

page 22

WHICH TWO ARE IDENTICAL?:

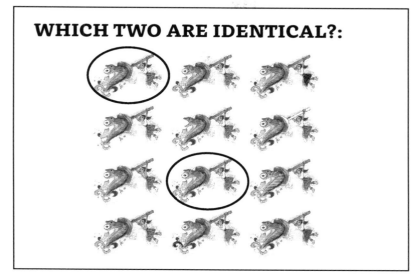

page 23

NAME THE PARTS

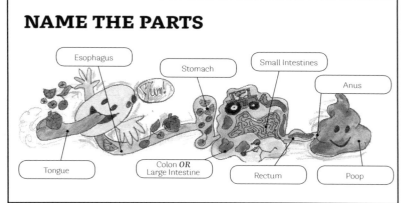

page 24

MAZE:

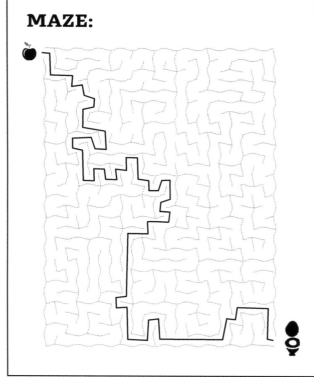

page 25

CHANGE ONE LETTER:

month > mouth
phew > chew
tenth > teeth
jelly > belly
color > colon
rectus > rectum
ants > anus
toiler > toilet

RHYME IT!: CHEW

Possible rhymes: blew, blue, brew, clue, coo, coup, crew, cue, do, due, drew, ewe, few, flew, flu, glue, gnu, goo, grew, hue, hew, knew, lieu, new, pew, queue, rue, shoe, shrew, skew, slew, spew, stew, threw, through, to, too, view, two true, whew, who, woo, yew, you, zoo

page 26

WORDFINDER: Possible words in INTESTINES:

2-letter words: in, is, it

3-letter words: inn, tin, tie, nit, set, sit, net, tee, sin, see, ten, its

4-letter words: ties, nets, nest, tens, inns, test, sees, tent, tees, nine, snit, sins, tint, teen, seen, sets, sent, tins, sits, site, tine, sine

5-letter words: tents, tins, tests, tenet, sense, stint, teens, snits, sites, tense, nests, inset

6-letter words: tenses, intent, insets, tennis, insist, tenets, testes

7-letter words: intense, tensest, intents, tiniest

page 27

UNCOVER A MESSAGE:

In your rectum

page 30

MATCH THE SHADOW

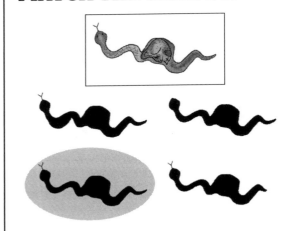

page 31

WORDFINDER:

Possible words in RECTUM:

3-letter words: cue, rum, rut, met, emu, rue, cut

4-letter words: cute, cure, term, curt, true, ecru, mute

Possible words in STRETCHED:

5-letter words: teeth, retch, heeds, shred, sheet, sheer, steed, reeds, steer, reset, herds, these, three, crest, creed, chest, cheer, there, deter, erect, terse

6-letter words: street, detest, detect, desert, tether, etched, tested, secret, cheers, rested, screed, setter

page 32

GUESSING GAME:

1. **b)** Your stomach is about the size of a grapefruit.

2. **a)** Your colon is about 3 feet (1 meter) long.

3. **c)** Your small intestine is about 22 feet long (7 meters).

4. **a)** It takes about 7 seconds for food to get from your mouth to your stomach.

5. **b)** It takes 6-8 hours for food to travel from your stomach through your small intestine.

page 36

WHICH IS IDENTICAL?:

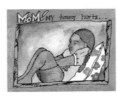
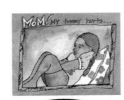
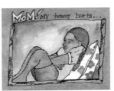
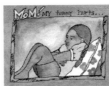
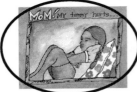
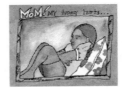

page 37

page 37

DECODE THE MESSAGE:
Just do your best

WORDFINDER: Possible words in ENEMA:
2-letter words: me, an, ma, am
3-letter words: men, man
4-letter words: name, mean, mane, amen

page 38

FIND THE DIFFERENCES:

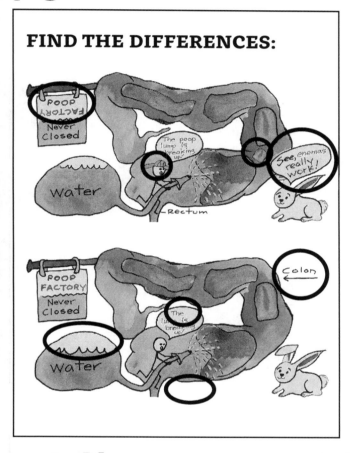

page 39

WHICH TWO ARE IDENTICAL?:

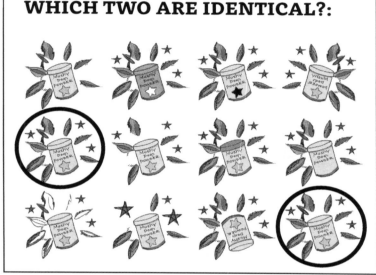

page 40

DECODE THE MESSAGE:
Right after you eat

page 41

WORD SCRAMBLE:
1) stool
2) forward
3) knees
4) apart

page 42

WORD SEARCH: IN THE WOODS

```
Q K A Y L U V C Z G C X U W E T Q S T Y
G J B T X M S C Z G O W L G F A Q F C W
J C F D W J X C W C R K B T N N C I C H
W Y G R C R U J O W O O D C H U K I R U
P Z S X O Z W R I Y Q U C I V K L Q I B
Q L T W J G W A W D O Y A H Y T A B C A
B W U Q J C P C U S H T T D A J Y D K D
M B O B C A T C W E A S E L G W X O E E
F E O W S U E O Y W G H R M L W K R T T
J M A P S F N O S G S X P C A O O M Y Q
G P Z G P Z Y N T S W B I H F O X O D Z
A O H A O S D B C Z I L I J D G U F K
C R E N L E S X O F V B L P N P R S H L
V C N Q X W T S U G K F A M D E O E W E
L U A I A T O V U R M R R U H C U O Z Z
L P Y O F F H S M N A B N X K N V V W
P I S C R O W H F P Y B C K W E D T M I
Z N Q V R A Y B I W M B B E A R H M T X
D E C H W B B S G Y B I M K U F O B A F
E M Q D D E E R M T E T W P I H G N O S
```

page 43

MAZE:

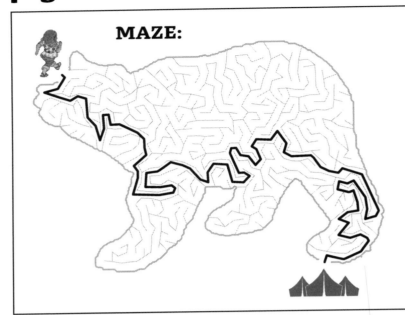

RHYME IT! STOOL
Possible rhymes:

cool, cruel, drool, dual, fool, fuel, ghoul, jewel, mule, pool, rule, school, spool, tool, yule

page 46

CROSSWORD:
FOLLOW YOUR FOOD

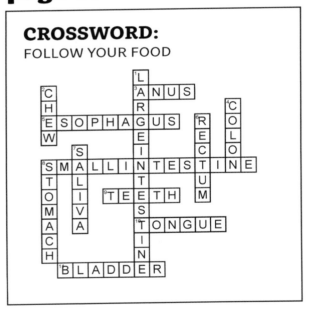

page 47

WHICH TWO ARE IDENTICAL?:

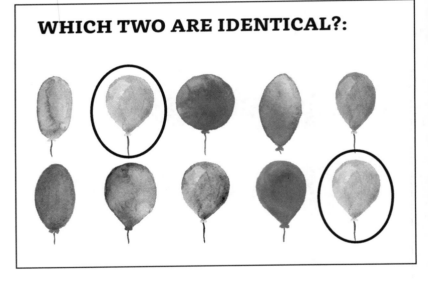

page 48

WORDFINDER: Possible words in BLADDER:
2-letter words: ad, be
3-letter words: lad, lab, are, red, ale, led, rad, add, era, bad, bar, bed, ear, dad, dab, bra
4-letter words: bred, read, real, drab, earl, dear, dead, lard, dare, lead, bale, bald, bard, bare, bead, bear, able, bled, deal
5-letter words: blare, dared, bared, blade, bread, beard, dread, addle, alder

RHYME IT!:

BLADDER
Possible rhymes:
ladder, madder, sadder

page 49

MAZE:

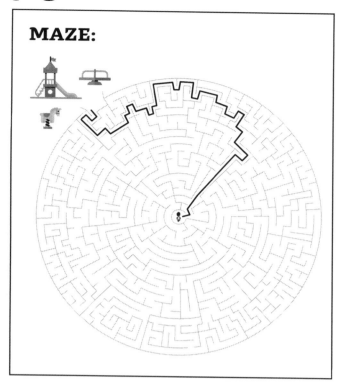

page 50

WHICH TWO ARE IDENTICAL?:

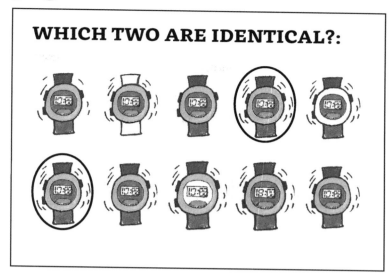

page 51

FIND THE DIFFERENCES:

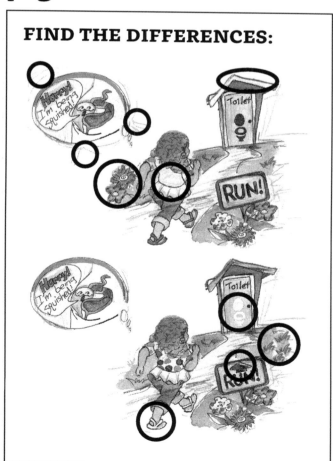

page 52

MAZE:

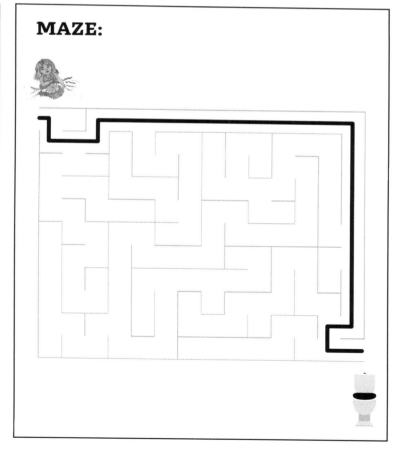

page 54 & 55

WORD SEARCH: ALL OVER THE WORLD

BEGINNER

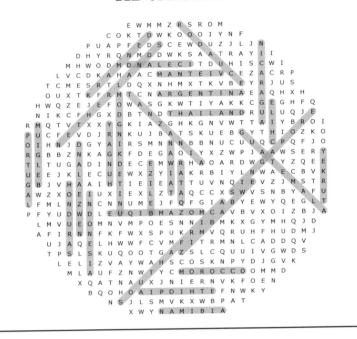

ADVANCED

page 56

WORDFINDER:

Possible words in ENURESIS:

2-letter words: us, in, is

3-letter words: sue, sun, urn, use, sin, rue, run, see, sir, ire

4-letter words: sine, user, urns, sure, sire, sere, rise, ruin, seen, seer, ruse

5-letter words: reuse, rinse, sense, risen, resin, issue, sneer, inure, urine, ensue, siren, reins, sinus, nurse

6-letter words: series, ensure

7-letter words: reissue, sunrise

page 57

WHICH TWO ARE IDENTICAL?:

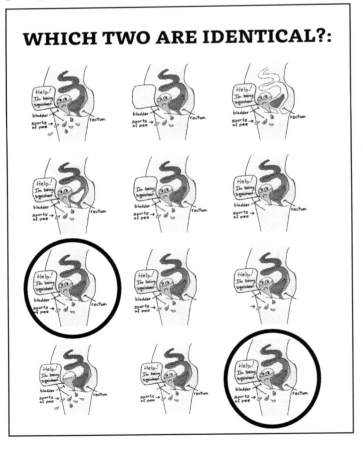

page 58

RHYME IT!: SHRINK
Possible rhymes: blink, brink, clink, drink, fink, ink, kink, link, mink, pink, sink, skink, slink, stink, sync, think, wink, zinc

page 59

WHAT DID DR. POOPER SAY?

Right after you eat

page 60

RHYME IT!: FLOPPY
Possible rhymes: copy, poppy, choppy, sloppy

page 61

WORDFINDER: Possible words in ENCOPRESIS:

2-letter words: or, no, so, in, on, is
3-letter words: pee, son, pin, con, pie, per, cop, pen, pro, ice, one, rip, nip, see, nor, ire, ion, sip, sir, eon, sin, ore
4-letter words: seep, seen, epic, icon, see, iron, cope, cons, cone, coin, spin, crop, snip, corn, core, sore, ones, peon, rise, once, ripe, open, rice, peer, pier, nope, nice, pore, rose, ripe, rope, nose, pose
5-letter words: spice, price, scorn, press, poser, spine, score, spire, sneer, snipe, since, rinse, ripen, scene, scope, prose, sense, snore, scone, prone, poise, cross, opine, creep, crepe, crisp, piece, niece, noise
6-letter words: screen, nosier, person, prince, recipe, reopen, pierce, opener, prison, recess, corpse, censor, copier, sensor, senior, encore
7-letter words: process, sincere, pioneer, precise, species
8-letter words: princess, response

page 62

WHICH TWO ARE IDENTICAL?:

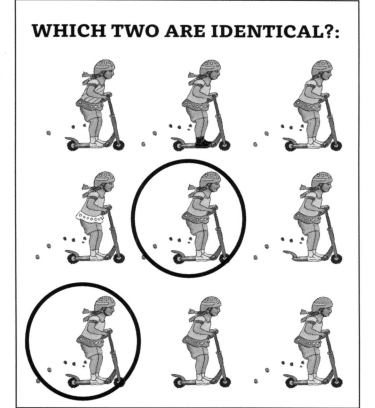

page 63

DECODE THE MESSAGE:

I need to pee

page 64

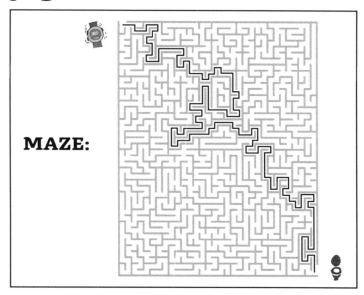

MAZE:

page 65

WORDFINDER:

Possible words in BATHROOM:
2-letter words: am, at, to, ma, oh, ah, ha
3-letter words: rat, ram, tar, orb, tab, rot, rob, too, hat, ham, boa, bat, bar, art, arm, hot, mar, oar, oat, mob, mat
4-letter words: harm, hoot, oath, moot, moat, roam, math, mart, room, root, moth, boot, boar, atom, bath, tram, tomb, boat, boom, brat, both
5-letter words: throb, booth, robot, taboo, abhor, broom, motor, broth

page 66

MYSTERY WORDS:
Use Soap

UNSCRAMBLED WORDS: flush, soap, pee, skin, poop, toilet paper, paper towel

RHYME IT!: SINK
Possible rhymes:
sink: brink, blink, clink, drink, fink, ink, kink, mink, pink, rink, shrink, sink, slink, stink, sync, think, wink, zinc

page 67

WHICH TWO ARE IDENTICAL?:

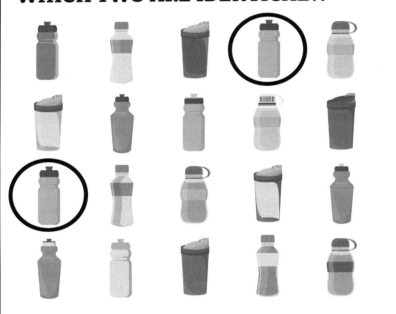

page 68

FIND THE DIFFERENCES:

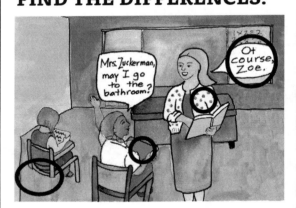

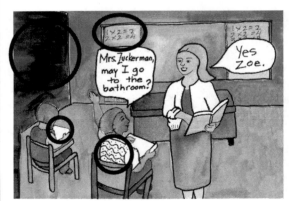

page 69

WORD SCRAMBLE:
cucumber, avocado, tomato, olive, pumpkin

page 70

WORD SEARCH:
A FRUITFUL SEARCH

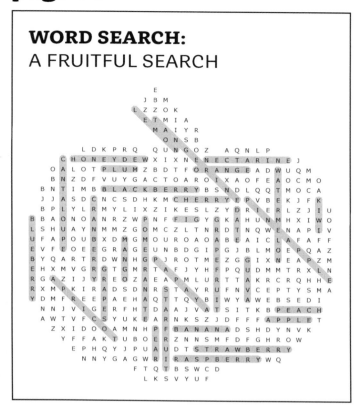

page 71

WHICH TWO ARE IDENTICAL?:

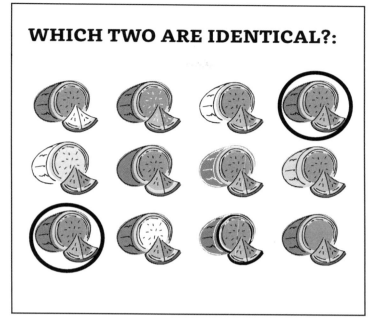

page 72

WORDFINDER:

Possible words in SPINACH:

2-letter words: as, is, in, an, ha, hi, ah

3-letter words: sin, his, ash, sip, sap, can, nap, pan, nip, pin, hip, cap

4-letter words: shin, pain, snip, spin, scan, snap, span, cash, ship, chin, inch, chip, chap

5-letter words: chain, china, panic, pinch

page 73

CROSSWORD:
GO GREEN!

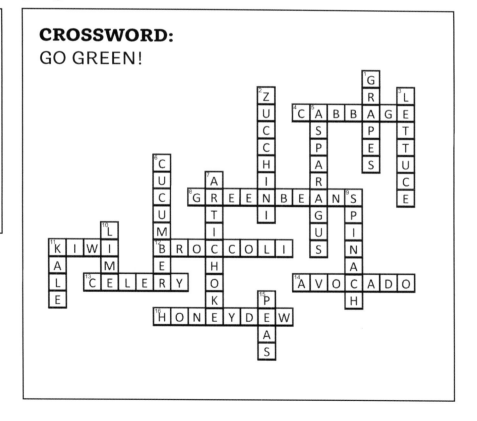

page 74

MAZE:

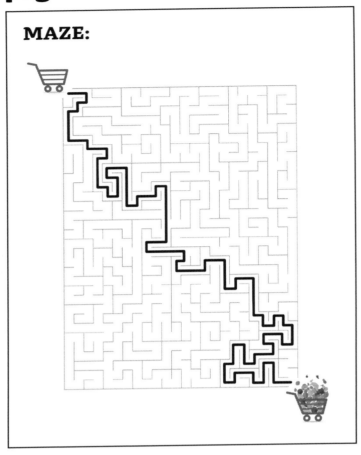

page 76

WORDFINDER:

Possible words in GARBANZO:

2-letter words: go, an, no, or, on

3-letter words: rob, ran, nab, nob, rag, orb, nor, oar, nag, gob, ban, bag, ago, bar, bog, boa, bra, gab

4-letter words: grab, boar, rang, born, garb, brag, bran, barn, bang

5-letter words: organ, baron, groan

page 79

MAZE:

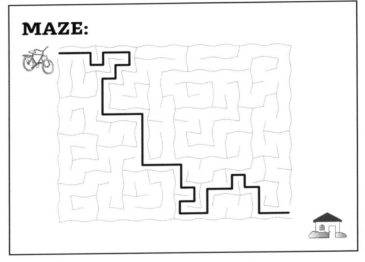

page 77

WORD SEARCH:
BEANS, BEANS, BEANS!

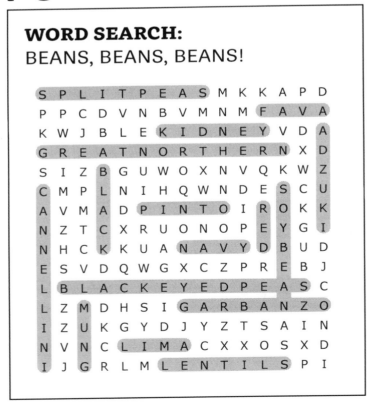

page 80

WORD SEARCH: GET MOVING!

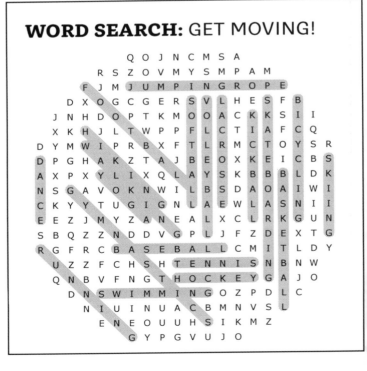

page 81

WHICH TWO ARE IDENTICAL?:

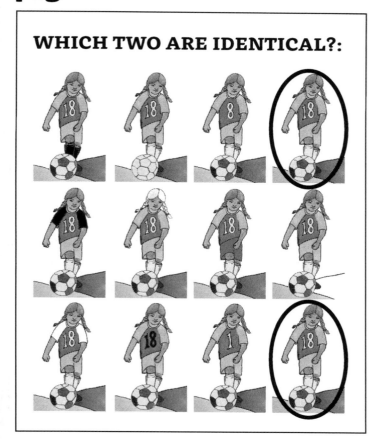

page 84

MAZE:

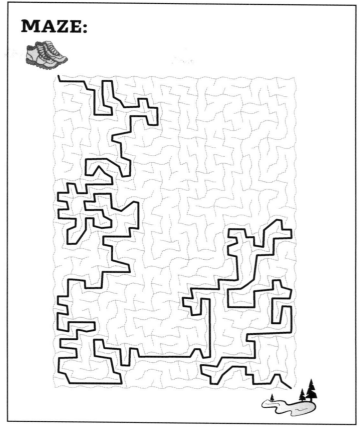

page 85

UNCOVER A MESSAGE:
running, basketball, soccer

RHYME IT!:

DANCE
Possible rhymes:
chance, glance, lance, manse, prance, stance, trance

JUMP
Possible rhymes:
bump, chump, clump, dump, grump, hump, plump, pump, rump, slump, stump, sump, thump

page 86

WORDFINDER:
Possible words in SCOOTER:
2-letter words: to, so, or
3-letter words: coo, set, toe, too, cot, rot, ore
4-letter words: rote, rose, root, tore, toes, sort, sore, soot, sect, cost, core, rest
5-letter words: score, torso, roost, score, scoot, crest
6-letter words: corset, escort, sector

Possible words in KICKBALL:
3-letter words: lab, ill, ilk, ick, cab, all, ail
4-letter words: lack, lick, call, kick, bill, bilk, back, bail, kill, balk, ball
5-letter words: black, lilac